Giampiero Ausili Cefaro · Carlos A. Perez · Domenico Genovesi
Annamaria Vinciguerra (Eds.)

A Guide for Delineation of Lymph Nodal Clinical Target Volume in Radiation Therapy

Giampiero Ausili Cefaro · Carlos A. Perez
Domenico Genovesi · Annamaria Vinciguerra
(Eds.)

A Guide for Delineation of Lymph Nodal Clinical Target Volume in Radiation Therapy

With 184 Figures and 12 Tables

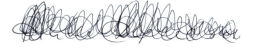

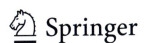

Giampiero Ausili Cefaro, MD
Department of Radiation Oncology
"G. d'Annunzio" University School
of Medicine
Chieti
Italy

Carlos A. Perez, MD
Department of Radiation Oncology
Washington University
St. Louis, MO
USA

Domenico Genovesi, MD
Department of Radiation Oncology
University Hospital
Chieti
Italy

Annamaria Vinciguerra, MD
Department of Radiation Oncology
University Hospital
Chieti
Italy

Translation from the Italian edition:
"Guida per la contornazione dei linfonodi in radioterapia".
First edition: October 2006
© 2006 Il Pensiero Scientifico Editore
All rights reserved in all countries
ISBN 88-490-0173-8

ISBN 978-3-540-77043-5	e-ISBN 978-3-540-77044-2

DOI 10.1007/978-3-540-77044-2

Library of Congress Control Number: 2008927198

© 2008 Il Pensiero Scientifico Editore

This work is subject to copyright. All rights are reserved, whether the whole or part of the material is concerned, specifically the rights of translation, reprinting, reuse of illustrations, recitation, broadcasting, reproduction on microfilm or in any other way, and storage in data banks. Duplication of this publication or parts thereof is permitted only under the provisions of the German Copyright Law of September 9, 1965, in its current version, and permission for use must always be obtained from the copyright holder. Violations are liable to prosecution under the German Copyright Law.

The use of general descriptive names, registered names, trademarks, etc. in this publication does not imply, even in the absence of a specific statement, that such names are exempt from the relevant protective laws and regulations and therefore free for general use.

Product liability: the publishers cannot guarantee the accuracy of any information about dosage and application contained in this book. In every individual case the user must check such information by consulting the relevant literature.

Cover design: Frido Steinen-Broo, eStudio Calamar, Spain
Production & Typesetting: le-tex publishing services oHG, Leipzig, Germany

Printed on acid-free paper

9 8 7 6 5 4 3 2

Springer.com

To our patients

Preface

Image-guided 3D Conformal or Intensity Modulated Radiation Therapy aims to deliver high doses of radiation to the tumor, while trying to maintain dose levels to healthy tissue within tolerable limits. Therefore, it is of key importance to define the different target volumes, gross tumor volume (GTV), clinical target volume (CTV), planning target volume (PTV), and organs at risk (OARs), on the basis of in-depth knowledge of the human anatomy, of anatomicoradiological aspects, and of anatomical and geometric variations during the radiation planning and treatment.

We have prepared this guide to meet the needs of radiation oncologists: our intention is to provide them with guidelines for identifying and defining the lymph node structures to be included in the treatment plan. Meeting this need also implies responding to findings in the literature, which, as regards lymph node structures, reveal differences in contouring practices not only among different radiotherapy centers, but also, quite often, among radiation oncologists working in the same center.

The book, after providing a brief anatomical description of the human lymphatic system, reviews the main anatomical classifications which take into account lymph drainage pathways in the various regions and describe the progression pathways of the various types of cancer. We use well-established classifications for the head and neck region and the mediastinum, while we employ more recent or still evolving classifications for the abdominal and pelvic regions. We also provide reference tables that facilitate the identification of the lymph nodes described by the various classification systems, which might be hard to find in scans performed without contrast medium.

Together with experienced radiologists for each anatomical region, we have developed a set of standards for the acquisition of planning CT images, standardizing the parameters for scan performance and those concerning patient positioning and immobilization.

In the second section of the book we describe the role and importance of radiological imaging in target definition, including lymph nodes, especially for image-guided radiation therapy (IGRT).

In the third section, radiologists and radiation oncologists have identified and defined the lymph nodes in the planning CT scans, concurrently identifying and numbering anatomical landmarks. Consultation of the CT images reproduced in this book, starting from the head and neck region down to the pelvic region, is facilitated by a flipping page which makes it possible to read the anatomicoradiological tables while viewing the scans.

While we are fully aware that our work is far from having resolved all the issues of lymph nodal area identification, including taking into account the variability of each patient's physical shape, we hope it will prove to be a useful tool for young and, if we may venture, also for not-so-young radiation oncologists and be an appropriate support in the delicate phase of radiation treatment planning.

Giampiero Ausili Cefaro
Carlos A. Perez
Domenico Genovesi
Annamaria Vinciguerra

Contents

Section I
General Considerations ... 1

1 Anatomy ... 3
1.1 Head and Neck Region ... 3
1.1.1 Occipital Lymph Nodes ... 3
1.1.2 Mastoid or Retroauricular Lymph Nodes ... 3
1.1.3 Parotid Lymph Nodes ... 4
1.1.4 Submandibular Lymph Nodes ... 4
1.1.5 Submental Lymph Nodes ... 4
1.1.6 Facial Lymph Nodes ... 5
1.1.7 Sublingual Lymph Nodes ... 5
1.1.8 Retropharyngeal Lymph Nodes ... 5
1.1.9 Anterior Cervical Lymph Nodes ... 5
1.1.10 Lateral Cervical Lymph Nodes ... 5
1.2 Thoracic Region ... 6
1.2.1 Parietal Lymph Nodes ... 6
1.2.2 Visceral Lymph Nodes ... 7
1.3 Upper Abdominal Region ... 7
1.3.1 Abdominal Visceral Lymph Nodes ... 8
1.3.2 Lumboaortic Lymph Nodes ... 8
1.4 Pelvic Region ... 8
1.4.1 Group of the Common Iliac Lymph Nodes ... 8
1.4.2 Group of the Internal Iliac Lymph Nodes (or Hypogastric) ... 9
1.4.3 Group of the External Iliac Lymph Nodes ... 9
1.4.4 Sacral or Presacral Lymph Nodes ... 10
1.4.5 Inguinal Lymph Nodes ... 10

2 Lymph Node Classification ... 11
2.1 Head and Neck Region ... 11
2.2 Mediastinal Region ... 13
2.3 Upper Abdominal Region ... 20
2.4 Pelvic Region ... 26

3 Anatomicoradiological Boundaries ... 29
3.1 Head and Neck Region ... 29
3.2 Mediastinal Region ... 30
3.3 Upper Abdominal Region ... 34
3.4 Pelvic Region ... 34

4 Planing CT: Technical Notes ... 39

Section II
Target Volume Delineation in Modern Radiation Therapy ... 43

5 Critical Importance of Target Definition, Including Lymph Nodes, in Image-Guided Radiation Therapy ... 45
5.1 Target Volume and Critical Structure Delineation ... 47
5.2 Delineation of Lymph Node Volumes ... 53

5.3	Implications of Target Definition for Innovative Technology in Contemporary Radiation Therapy	... 56		7	Mediastinal Lymph Nodes	97
5.4	Quality Assurance	56		8	Upper Abdominal Region Lymph Nodes	113
5.5	Cost Benefit and Utility	57				
5.6	Conclusions	59		9	Pelvic Lymph Nodes	137
				10	Digitally Reconstructed Radiographs (DRRs)	161

Section III
Axial CT Radiological Anatomy 61

6 Head and Neck Lymph Nodes 63

References 163

Contributors

Antonietta Augurio, MD
Department of Radiation Oncology
University Hospital
Chieti
Italy

Nicola Filippo Basilico, MD
Department of Radiation Oncology
University Hospital
Chieti
Italy

Raffaella Basilico, MD
Department of Radiology
University Hospital
Chieti
Italy

Marco D'Alessandro, MD
Department of Radiation Oncology
University Hospital
Chieti
Italy

Angelo Di Pilla, MD
Department of Radiation Oncology
University Hospital
Chieti
Italy

Antonella Filippone, MD
Department of Radiology
University Hospital
Chieti
Italy

James A. Purdy, PhD
Department of Radiation Oncology
University of California, Davis Medical Center
Sacramento, CA
USA

Pietro Sanpaolo, MD
Department of Radiation Oncology
Regional Oncological Hospital, CROB
Rionero in Vulture
Italy

Maria Luigia Storto, MD
Director of Radiology Department
"G. d'Annunzio" University School of Medicine
Chieti
Italy

Maria Taraborrelli, MD
Department of Radiation Oncology
University Hospital
Chieti
Italy

Armando Tartaro
Professor of Radiology
"G. d'Annunzio" University School of Medicine
Chieti
Italy

Lucia Anna Ursini, MD
Department of Radiation Oncology
University Hospital
Chieti
Italy

Section I

General Considerations

Anatomy

1.1 Head and Neck Region

The head and neck region [1, 2] has a dense lymphatic network which, through the jugular, spinal accessory, and transverse cervical nodes under the jugular-subclavian axis, drains lymph from the skull base to the thoracic duct.

Lymph drainage of the anatomical structures belonging to this region is ipsilateral, apart from tonsil, soft palate, basal tongue, posterior pharyngeal wall, and, especially, nasopharynx, all of which drain bilaterally. Vocal folds, paranasal sinuses, and middle ear do not have lymph vessels, or have them in limited number.

According to Rouvière, head and neck lymph nodes are clustered in groups or form chains that are satellites of the main blood vessels (Fig. 1.1). These nodal groups are listed below:
- The **pericervical ring**, which includes six nodal groups surrounding the upper neck:
  - Occipital nodes
  - Mastoid or retroauricular nodes
  - Parotid nodes
  - Submandibular nodes
  - Submental nodes
  - Facial nodes
- **Sublingual** and **retropharyngeal lymph nodes**, located medial to the pericervical nodal ring
- **Anterior** and **lateral cervical lymph nodes of the neck**, located anterior and lateral to the neck, respectively

1.1.1 Occipital Lymph Nodes

They are adjacent to the occipital artery. Rouvière distinguishes them into **superficial**, **subfascial**, and **submuscular**.

The superficial nodes are located at the level of the insertion of the sternocleidomastoid and the trapezius muscles; the subfascial nodes are situated above the splenius muscle; and the submuscular nodes are located below the splenius muscle.

They receive lymphatics from the occipital area of the scalp and from the skin and deep regions of the upper nape.

1.1.2 Mastoid or Retroauricular Lymph Nodes

They are located on the superficial aspect of the anterior and superior insertions of the sternocleidomastoid muscle.

They receive lymphatics from the skin of the medial aspect of the ear, the back of the temporal region, and the parietal area of the skull.

A Guide for Delineation of Lymph Nodal Clinical Target Volume in Radiation Therapy

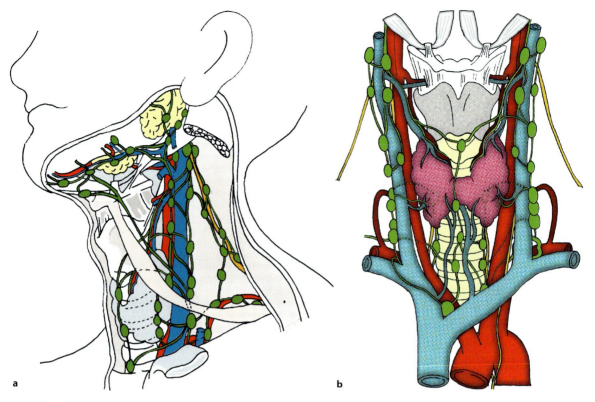

FIG. 1.1 a,b Main head and neck nodes. **a** Lateral view. **b** Anteroposterior view

1.1.3 Parotid Lymph Nodes

They are divided into:
- **Superficial nodes**. They are located in front of the tragus, along the superficial temporal vessels.
- **Extraglandular subfascial nodes**. They are located in the parotid cavity immediately below the fascia.
- **Deep intraglandular nodes**. They are scattered within the parotid gland, close to the external jugular vein and the facial nerve.

They receive lymphatics from the parotid, the frontal and temporal regions, lacrimal gland, upper eyelid, lateral half of the lower eyelid, tympanic membrane, Eustachian tube, auricle, external auditory meatus, nose, upper lip, cheek, and gums in the molar area.

1.1.4 Submandibular Lymph Nodes

These are deep nodes, anatomically located in the submandibular cavity, adjacent to the salivary gland and the anterior facial vein. Rouvière divided them into five groups: periglandular, perivascular, retrovascular, retroglandular, and intracapsular.

They receive lymph collectors from the lower lip, lateral chin, cheek, gums, teeth, internal eyelids, anterior tongue, submandibular gland, sublingual gland, and floor of mouth.

1.1.5 Submental Lymph Nodes

They are located superficially at the level of the suprahyoid region, on the lower aspect of the mylohyoid muscle.

They drain the chin, lower lip, cheeks, gums, lower incisors, floor of mouth, and tip of tongue.

1.1.6 Facial Lymph Nodes

They are located along the course of the facial lymph vessels, which follow the facial artery and vein; they include the buccinator, mandibular, infraorbital, and zygomatic nodes which receive lymphatics from adjacent areas.

1.1.7 Sublingual Lymph Nodes

These are inconstant and are located along the course of the collector vessels of the tongue.

1.1.8 Retropharyngeal Lymph Nodes

They are distinguished into **medial**, located along the lymphatics of the posterior aspect of the pharynx, above the hyoid bone, and **lateral**, at the level of the lateral masses of the atlas, in contact with the lateral margin of the posterior pharyngeal wall.

They receive lymph from the nasal cavity, paranasal sinuses, palate, middle ear, nasopharynx, and oropharynx.

1.1.9 Anterior Cervical Lymph Nodes

They are located below the hyoid bone, between the two vascular-nervous bundles of the neck. They are divided into two groups:
1. **Anterior jugular chain**. It is located below the superficial cervical fascia along the course of the anterior jugular vein.
2. **Juxtavisceral lymph nodes**. They are located frontal to the larynx (prelaryngeal), the thyroid (prethyroid), and the trachea (pretracheal), and on the lateral aspects of the trachea (recurrent chains). They drain larynx, thyroid, trachea, and esophagus.

1.1.10 Lateral Cervical Lymph Nodes

They are divided into:
- **Superficial** (external jugular chain). They follow the external jugular vein.
- **Deep**. They are located in the carotid region and the supraclavicular cavity. They extend posteriorly under the trapezius muscle, while downward and forward they reach below the clavicle to the anterior chest. According to Rouvière's classification three chains are distinguished:
  1. **Internal jugular chain**, satellite of the vein: it includes an anterior and a lateral group. The anterior lymph nodes run anterior to the jugular vein, while the lateral ones follow the lateral wall of the vein, extending from the posterior belly of the digastric muscle to the crossing of the omohyoid muscle passing behind the vein in the lower portion. The internal jugular chain drains the anterior portion of the head and neck, nasal cavity, pharynx, ear, tongue, palate, salivary glands, tonsils, and thyroid.
  2. **Spinal accessory nerve chain**: it follows the lateral branch of the nerve in the posterior triangle of the neck. It runs under the trapezius muscle, starting from the posterior margin of the sternocleidomastoid muscle to the upper margin of the supraspinous fossa. It receives lymph from the occipital, postauricular, and suprascapular nodes and from the posterior and lateral nape, lateral neck, and shoulder.
  3. **Transverse chain of the neck** (supraclavicular): it follows the transverse artery. It is located transversally, from the lower margin of the spinal accessory chain to the junction of the internal jugular and subclavian veins. It receives lymph from the accessory spinal chain, the breast region, the anterior and lateral neck, and the upper limb.

1.2 Thoracic Region

Thoracic lymph nodes [3] are divided into parietal and visceral.

1.2.1 Parietal Lymph Nodes

- **Internal thoracic lymph nodes**. They form two chains, on either side of the posterior aspect of the sternum, from the xiphoid process to the first rib, along the course of the internal thoracic vessels. They receive lymph collectors from the skin of the anterior thoracic wall, the anterior intercostal spaces, the epigastric area, the medial breast, and the anterior diaphragmatic lymph nodes.
- **Intercostal lymph nodes**. They are located in the posterior portion of intercostal spaces, near the heads of the ribs; they are also called paravertebral nodes. They drain lymphatic vessels from the thoracic wall, which receive lymph from the parietal pleura and from the lymphatic vessels of the spinal cord and paravertebral grooves.
- **Diaphragmatic lymph nodes**. Located in the diaphragmatic convexity, they are grouped in the loose cellular tissue at the base of the pericardium. They are divided into an anterior group, behind the xiphoid process; a right lateral group at the level of the diaphragmatic orifice of the inferior vena cava; a left lateral group, near the phrenic nerve; and a posterior group behind the diaphragmatic crura. They receive lymphatic vessels from the diaphragm.

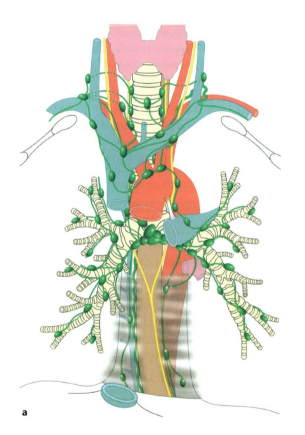
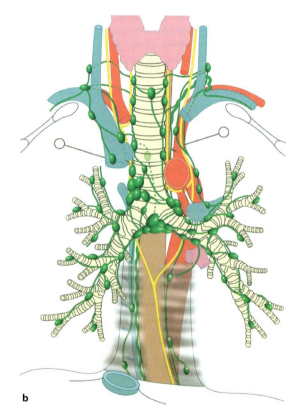

FIG. 1.2 a,b Main visceral mediastinal nodes. **a** Superficial view. **b** Deep view

1.2.2 Visceral Lymph Nodes

Rouvière divided the visceral lymph nodes of the chest into four groups (Fig. 1.2):
1. **Anterior mediastinal or prevascular nodes.** They run between the sternum and the heart, anterior to the great vessels. They receive lymphatics from the thymus, heart, and trachea.
2. **Posterior mediastinal or juxtaesophageal nodes.** They are located between the posterior aspect of the pericardium and the vertebral column: they are divided into pre- and retroesophageal nodes. They drain the lateral and posterior lymph nodes and the esophagus.
3. **Peritracheobronchial lymph nodes.** They are very numerous and are located around the trachea and main bronchi. They receive lymphatic vessels from the lungs and heart. They are divided into:
   - **Lymph nodes of the pulmonary pedicle**, located between the origin of the bronchus and the mediastinal pleural reflection
   - **Subcarinal nodes**, situated below the carina
   - **Peritracheal nodes**, located on the anterior and lateral aspects of the trachea and a few posteriorly
4. **Intrapulmonary lymph nodes.** They follow the bronchial divisions in the lungs.

1.3 Upper Abdominal Region

Abdominal lymph nodes [1, 3, 4] can be divided into two main groups: visceral nodes and lumboaortic nodes (Fig. 1.3).

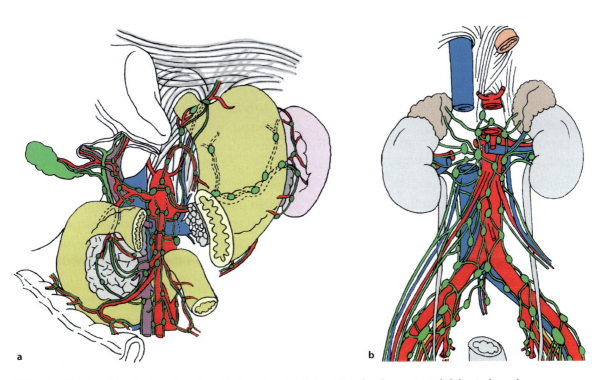

FIG. 1.3 a,b Main abdominal lymph nodes. **a** Perigastric region. **b** Lymph nodes along principal abdominal vessels

1.3.1 Abdominal Visceral Lymph Nodes

Important lymph node chains are grouped along the lymphatic pathways from the abdominal organs:
- **Coronary chain** (left gastric lymph nodes). It runs along the lesser gastric curvature and the left gastric artery.
- **Gastroepiploic chain** (right gastric lymph nodes) along the greater gastric curvature.
- **Splenic or lienal chain** (pancreaticolienal chain) along the upper pancreas and at the hilum of spleen.
- **Hepatic chain** (hepatic lymph nodes). It runs along the hepatic artery and the retropancreatic common bile duct.
- **Superior and inferior mesenteric chains.** They run between the mesenteric layers. The lymph nodes of these chains are especially numerous at the level of the jejunum where they run along the course of the branches of the mesenteric artery and the root of the mesentery.

1.3.2 Lumboaortic Lymph Nodes

They can be divided into eight subgroups according to their position with respect to the aorta and the vena cava. Below, we list the subgroups of the nodes located around the aorta.
- **Lateroaortic group** (bilateral). The right lateroaortic subgroup can be further divided into: aortocaval, lateral caval, precaval, and postcaval subgroups, all adjacent to the vena cava. Lateroaortic lymph nodes receive afferents from the common iliac lymph nodes and the lumbar, spermatic, and utero-ovarian lymphatics.
- **Preaortic group**. These nodes are located anterior to the aorta, immediately below the origin of the superior and inferior mesenteric arteries, and they receive afferent lymphatics from the rectum, colon, small intestine, pancreas, stomach, liver, and spleen.
- **Postaortic group**. These nodes are located posterior to the aorta and anterior to the third-fourth lumbar vertebrae.

1.4 Pelvic Region

Lymphatic drainage of the pelvis [1, 3, 4] is commonly divided into two chains: parietal and visceral. The parietal lymphatics include the lymphatic vessels of the skin and the superficial fascia of the anterior and posterior pelvic walls. The visceral lymphatic chains include the lymphatic vessels draining the urogenital region, the rectum, and the peritoneum.

In addition to the lymph nodes situated in strictly visceral locations, the pelvic visceral lymph nodes also comprise the following groups of nodes (Fig. 1.4) [5].

1.4.1 Group of the Common Iliac Lymph Nodes

It consists of three nodal chains:
1. Lateral
2. Intermediate
3. Medial

The **lateral chain** is an extension of the lateral chain of external iliac nodes and is located lateral to the common iliac artery. The **intermediate chain** consists of the nodes of the lumbosacral fossa, which is delimited anteriorly by the common iliac vessels, laterally by the psoas muscle, medially by the lumbosacral vertebrae and posteriorly/inferiorly by the ala of sacrum. The lymph nodes can be located between the common iliac artery and veins. The **medial chain** is located in the triangular area formed by the two common iliac arteries, from the aortic bifurcation to the bifurcation of the internal and external iliac arteries. The lymph nodes of the sacral promontory are included in this chain.

The common iliac lymph nodes receive afferents

Anatomy

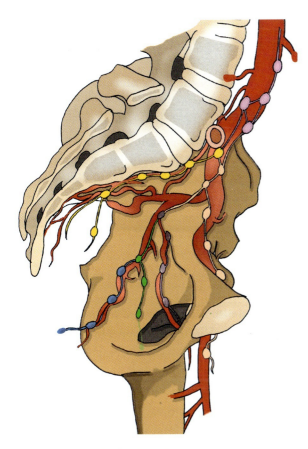

FIG. 1.4 Main pelvic lymph nodes

from the internal and external iliac nodes, presacral nodes, and some lymphatics coming directly from pelvic viscera. The lymphatics of the common iliac nodes ascend toward the para-aortic nodes.

1.4.2 Group of the Internal Iliac Lymph Nodes (or Hypogastric)

The internal iliac nodes include several nodal chains which run along the various visceral branches of the internal iliac artery, such as the uterine artery, the prostatic branches of the inferior and middle rectal arteries, the superior and inferior gluteal arteries, and the internal pudendal artery. These nodes are difficult to distinguish since they are adjacent to each other. However, we can distinguish two different nodal chains: the anterior nodes, located anterior to the hypogastric vessels near the origin of the umbilical and obturator arteries, and the lateral sacral nodes, located along the course of the lateral sacral arteries, anterior to the first and second sacral foramen.

The internal iliac nodes receive the gluteal and ischial lymphatics, the obturator lymphatics, and the visceral pelvic lymphatics (coming from rectum, bladder, prostate, seminal vesicles, deferent ducts, uterus, and vagina).

1.4.3 Group of the External Iliac Lymph Nodes

This group includes the lymph nodes located around the external iliac vessels, and includes three nodal chains:
1. Lateral
2. Intermediate
3. Medial

The **lateral chain** includes the nodes located lateral to the external iliac artery and medial to the psoas muscle. The **intermediate chain** includes the nodes located between the external iliac artery and veins. The **medial chain** includes the nodes located medial and posterior to the external iliac vein.

There are controversies concerning the denomination of the medial chain nodes, which are also known as obturator lymph nodes. These nodes are adjacent to the obturator vessels and, according to some authors, should not belong to the external iliac nodes, but rather to the internal iliac nodes. However, other authors [6] consider medial chain nodes as being functionally linked to the external iliac chain and located in an area delimited superiorly by the external iliac vein, posteriorly by the internal iliac artery followed by the pelvic ureter, and inferiorly by the obturator nerve. In surgical terminology they are referred to as obturator lymph nodes, but should not be confused with the small, isolated obturator lymph node located in the internal foramen of the obturator canal, in the lower portion of the homonymous fossa. This single lymph node is functionally linked to the internal iliac chain throughout its efferent vessels.

The external iliac nodes receive inguinal lymphatics, deep lymphatics from the anterior and subumbilical portion of the abdominal wall, circumflex iliac lymphatics, and part of the genitourinary lymphatics.

1.4.4 Sacral or Presacral Lymph Nodes

They are located in the anterior aspect of sacrum, on either side of the rectum. They drain lymphatics from the rectum and the pelvic wall.

1.4.5 Inguinal Lymph Nodes

The lymph nodes of the inguinofemoral region can be divided into superficial and deep nodes.

The **superficial inguinal nodes** are located in the subcutaneous tissue anterior to the inguinal ligament and run along the course of the superficial (distal) femoral vein and saphenous vein. They can be further subdivided into four areas indicated by two imaginary, vertical and horizontal lines crossing at the level of the saphenofemoral junction:
1. Upper lateral group
2. Upper medial group
3. Lower lateral group
4. Lower medial group

The lower medial and lower lateral nodes drain the superficial lymphatics from the lower limb. The upper lateral nodes receive superficial lymphatics from the lateral gluteal region and from the lateral and posterior subumbilical region of the abdominal wall. The upper medial nodes drain the external genitalia, the anus, the superficial perineum, the medial gluteal region, and the anterior subumbilical abdominal wall.

The **deep inguinal nodes** run along the common femoral vessels, within the femoral canal, medial to the femoral vein, and drain into the medial chain of external iliac nodes. They are separated from the group of superficial inguinal nodes by fascial planes which are not clearly visible on computed tomography (CT) images. The inguinal ligament at the origin of inferior epigastric vessels and circumflex iliac vessels is used as a landmark for distinguishing the deep inguinal nodes from the medial chain of the external iliac nodes.

The deep inguinal nodes drain lymphatics from the superficial inguinal lymph nodes, the glans, the clitoris, and some deep lymphatics of the lower limb.

Lymph Node Classification

The presence in our body of a rich network of lymph vessels and numerous lymph node stations prompted several authors to draw up classifications that would take into account lymph drainage pathways in the various districts and would be useful for describing tumor progression pathways.

The lymph node classifications of different anatomical regions, mostly prepared by surgeons, have provided valuable help for the execution and standardization of surgical procedures, offering an effective tool for ensuring their reproducibility.

With the development of new radiotherapy techniques, especially conformal radiotherapy, radiation oncologists have also started using these classifications to define the nodal clinical target volume (CTV) [7, 8] that appears to be increasingly selective.

We have considered the following classifications for lymph node contouring on CT:
- **Head and neck region,** classification of the American Head and Neck Society/American Academy of Otolaryngology Head and Neck Surgery (AHNS/AAO-HNS, 1998, Robbins classification).
- **Mediastinal region,** American Joint Committee on Cancer/International Union Against Cancer (AJCC/UICC) classification, 1996 (Mountain and Dresler).
- **Upper abdominal region,** classification of the Japanese Gastric Cancer Association (JGCA).
- **Pelvic region,** we referred to the distribution of lymph node groups relative to the main arteries.

2.1 Head and Neck Region

For nearly four decades, the most commonly used classification of cervical lymph nodes was that developed by Rouvière [2] in 1938, based on a previous classification by Trotter (1930) [9] which was based on an earlier study by Poirer and Charpy in 1909 [10]. This classification defined lymph node areas based on anatomical limits established through palpation or surgical dissection.

In subsequent years, the need was felt for a classification based on new clinical and pathophysiological considerations, specifically, in relation to surgical neck dissection techniques; consequently, several new classification systems were proposed [11–14].

In 1991 the AAO-HNS classified neck lymph nodes into levels, following a system originally proposed by the Memorial Sloan-Kettering Cancer Group (New York) [15]. This classification, also known as the Robbins classification [16], distinguishes six levels:
- **IA**, submental lymph nodes
- **IB**, submandibular lymph nodes
- **II**, upper jugular lymph nodes
- **III**, middle jugular lymph nodes
- **IV**, lower jugular lymph nodes

- **V**, posterior triangle lymph nodes
- **VI**, anterior compartment lymph nodes

It considers the lymph nodes that are removed during neck dissections. The lymph nodes that are not commonly removed, such as retropharyngeal, parotid, buccal, and occipital nodes, are not included in the Robbins classification. Subsequently, this classification was recommended by the UICC [17].

In 1992, in the TNM classification of malignant tumors, the division of the head and neck lymph nodes into 12 groups was proposed, based on the descriptions made by Rouvière [18]:

1. Submental nodes
2. Submandibular nodes
3. Upper jugular lymph nodes
4. Middle jugular lymph nodes
5. Lower jugular lymph nodes
6. Dorsal cervical nodes along the spinal accessory nerve
7. Supraclavicular nodes
8. Prelaryngeal and paratracheal nodes
9. Retropharyngeal nodes
10. Parotid nodes
11. Buccal nodes
12. Retroauricular and occipital nodes

In 1997, the fifth edition of the cancer staging handbook of the AJCC [19], introduced, in addition to the Robbins classification, a further level including the lymph nodes below the suprasternal notch. Although they are not located in the neck but in the upper mediastinum, lymph nodes belonging to this level can be involved in head and neck cancer (e.g., subglottic, hypopharyngeal, and thyroid tumors).

In 1998, 10 years after the start of the classification project, the AHNS in collaboration with the AAO-HNS, updated the original classification system of 1991 to account for the changes in head and neck cancer staging introduced by the AJCC [19]. K. Thomas Robbins headed the AHNS committee, whose members also included the radiologist Peter M. Som, who was tasked with defining the radiological margins of the various levels. The committee decided to continue using the six-level system (thus excluding the introduction of a level VII for upper mediastinal lymph nodes) and to indicate the lymph nodes through their anatomical sites (e.g., retropharyngeal, parotid, buccal, retroauricular, and suboccipital nodes). The main changes concerned the revision of the classification of neck dissections, and the proposal of a further subdivision of levels II and V into IIA–IIB, separated by the spinal accessory nerve, and VA–VB, divided by a plane defined by the inferior margin of the cricoid cartilage [20–23].

Each of these sublevels defines a site with a different clinical implication in the event of metastatic involvement. For instance, level II subclassification is justified by the fact that level IIB is mostly involved in oropharyngeal and nasopharyngeal tumors, while it is less often involved in neoplasms of the oral cavity, larynx, and hypopharynx. Thus, when tumors occur in the latter sites, without clinical involvement of sublevel IIA, it is not necessary to include level IIB in the dissection [20–23]. This is especially important if we consider the possible dysfunctions of the trapezius muscle due to manipulation of the spinal accessory nerve performed for removing level IIB nodes. Similar surgical considerations apply to level IA which is removed only in the presence of neoplasms of the floor of mouth, lips, anterior mobile tongue, or anterior alveolar mandibular arch. The subclassification into VA and VB is warranted by the fact that neoplasms that are the main cause of metastatic lymph nodes in those sites originate from the nasopharynx, the oropharynx, and skin structures of the posterior scalp for level VA, and from the thyroid for level VB (Fig. 2.1; Table 2.1).

Recently a group of authors [24] has proposed a further division of level VA into two sections, VAs

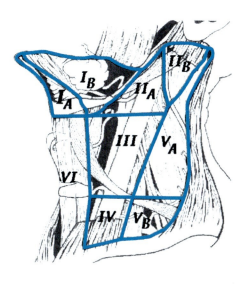

FIG. 2.1 Graphic representation of the six levels of lymph nodes according to the Robbins classification. Adapted from Robbins KT, Atkinson JLD, Byers RM, et al. (2001) [23]

(superior) and VAi (inferior), separated by a horizontal plane defined by the upper margin of the body of the hyoid bone, at the level of the lower two thirds of the spinal accessory nerve. The distinction between the posterior edge of sublevel IIB and the apex of sublevel VA is not clear, and is virtually impossible during most neck dissections. Indeed, for complete sublevel IIB removal, even the most experienced surgeons usually also remove the upper portion of sublevel VA. Already in 1987, Suen and Goepfert [25] had proposed inclusion of the apex of the portion that would be later defined sublevel VA, in sublevel IIB, thus considering that the upper edge of level V is adjacent to the lower part of the spinal accessory nerve.

Moreover, the upper part of sublevel VA only contains the superficial suprafascial occipital lymph nodes and, in smaller number, the subfascial and submuscular lymph nodes located close to the occipital insertion of the sternocleidomastoid muscle. These lymph nodes receive lymph drainage from the skin of the mastoid and occipital regions and are not usually involved in head and neck tumors, except in cases of skin cancer. In most head and neck carcinomas, dissection and/or radiation therapy [26] of the apex of level V are not necessary and should only be considered in some skin cancers of the posterior scalp and neck.

The same authors also introduced the division, considered by Robbins [20], of level IV into IVA (lymph nodes located deep into the sternal head of the sternocleidomastoid muscle) and IVB (deep into the clavicular head of the sternocleidomastoid muscle). In the past, Byers et al. [27] had also defined a level IIIB including lymph nodes situated far posterior to the internal jugular vein.

2.2 Mediastinal Region

Similar to the head and neck region, for the mediastinal region there are different classification systems which have been updated over the years.

In 1967, Rouvière [3] classified pulmonary lymph nodes dividing them into four groups:
1. Anterior mediastinal group
2. Posterior mediastinal group
3. Peritracheobronchial group
4. Intrapulmonary group

Table 2.1 – Robbins classification

Level	Name	Description	Regions drained
IA	Submental nodes	Lymph nodes within the triangular boundary of the anterior belly of the digastric muscles and the hyoid bone	Floor of mouth, anterior oral tongue, anterior mandibular alveolar ridge, and lower lip
IB	Submandibular nodes	Lymph nodes within the boundaries of the anterior and posterior bellies of the digastric muscle, the stylohyoid muscle, and the mandibular body. It includes the pre- and postglandular nodes and the pre- and postvascular nodes. The submandibular gland is included in the specimen when the lymph nodes within this triangle are removed	Oral cavity, anterior nasal cavity, and soft tissue structures of the midface, and submandibular gland
IIA–IIB	Upper jugular nodes	Lymph nodes located around the upper third of the internal jugular vein and adjacent to spinal accessory nerve extending from the level of the skull base to the level of the inferior border of the hyoid bone. The anterior (medial) boundary is the lateral border of the sternohyoid muscle and the stylohyoid muscle, and the posterior (lateral) boundary is the posterior border of the sternocleidomastoid muscle **IIA lymph nodes:** Lymph nodes located anterior (medial) to the vertical plane defined by the spinal accessory nerve **IIB lymph nodes:** Lymph nodes located posterior (lateral) to the vertical plane defined by the spinal accessory nerve	Oral cavity, nasal cavity, nasopharynx, oropharynx, hypopharynx, larynx, and parotid gland
III	Middle jugular nodes	Lymph nodes located around the middle third of the internal jugular vein extending from the inferior border of the hyoid bone to the inferior border of the cricoid bone. The anterior (medial) boundary is the lateral border of the sternohyoid muscle, and the posterior (lateral) boundary is the posterior border of the sternocleidomastoid muscle or the sensory branches of the cervical plexus	Oral cavity, nasopharynx, oropharynx, hypopharynx, and larynx
IV	Lower jugular nodes	Lymph nodes located around the lower third of the internal jugular vein extending from the inferior border of the cricoid bone to the clavicle. The anterior (medial) boundary is the lateral border of the sternohyoid muscle and the posterior (lateral) boundary is the posterior border of the sternocleidomastoid muscle or the sensory branches of the cervical plexus	Hypopharynx, cervical esophagus, and larynx
VA–VB	Posterior triangle nodes	This group is comprised predominantly of the lymph nodes located along the lower half of the spinal accessory nerve and the transverse cervical artery. The supraclavicular nodes are also included in this group. The superior boundary is formed by convergence of the sternocleidomastoid and trapezius muscles, the inferior boundary is the clavicle, the anterior (medial) boundary is the posterior border of the sternocleidomastoid muscle or the sensory branches of the cervical plexus, and the posterior (lateral) boundary is the anterior border of the trapezius muscle **VA lymph nodes:** Lymph nodes located above the horizontal plane defined by the inferior border of the cricoid cartilage. Included are the lymph nodes lying along the spinal accessory nerve **VB lymph nodes:** Lymph nodes located below the horizontal plane defined by the inferior border of the cricoid cartilage. Included are the lymph nodes lying along the transverse cervical artery and the supraclavicular nodes, except the Virchow node which is located in level IV	Nasopharynx and oropharynx
VI	Anterior compartment nodes	Lymph nodes in this compartment include the pre- and paratracheal nodes, precricoid (Delphian) node, and the perithyroidal nodes including the lymph nodes along the recurrent laryngeal nerves. The superior boundary is the hyoid bone, the inferior boundary is the suprasternal notch, and the lateral boundaries are the common carotid arteries	Thyroid gland, glottic and subglottic larynx, apex of the piriform sinus, and cervical esophagus

Source: Adapted from Robbins KT, Clayman G, Levine PA, et al. (2002) [22]

Subsequently, two main classifications were proposed: the classification of the AJCC adapted from Naruke [28–31] and that of the American Thoracic Society (ATS) and the Lung Cancer Study Group (LCSG) [32–36].

In 1978, Naruke suggested the use of an anatomical "map" in which the lymph node stations were numbered [29] and provided an anatomical definition of 14 lymph node stations:

1. Superior mediastinal lymph nodes, located at the upper third of the trachea within the thorax
2. Paratracheal lymph nodes, corresponding to a level between stations 1 and 4, and situated along the lateral sides of the trachea
3. Pretracheal, retrotracheal, or posterior mediastinal, and anterior mediastinal lymph nodes
4. Tracheobronchial nodes, in the lateral portion of the junction between the trachea and the main bronchi (on the right side they are located at the level of the azygos vein and on the left side they are adjacent to the subaortic lymph nodes)
5. Subaortic lymph nodes
6. Para-aortic lymph nodes
7. Subcarinal lymph nodes
8. Paraesophageal nodes (below carina)
9. Pulmonary ligament lymph nodes
10. Hilar lymph nodes
11. Interlobar lymph nodes (the right interlobar nodes are classified, if necessary, into superior and inferior)
12. Lobar lymph nodes
13. Segmental lymph nodes
14. Subsegmental lymph nodes

The Japan Lung Cancer Society adopted this mapping and published a handbook for the classification of lung cancer, providing detailed descriptions based on CT imaging and surgical findings, for each of the stations defined by Naruke. Although this manual has been widely used in Japan, it has not been universally accepted. One of the main reasons for its limited acceptance was the lack of an English translation until March 2000 [37].

The AJCC produced a classification of 13 lymph node stations [38], however, it did not provide a description of the anatomical boundaries of each station:

- **N2 nodes (within the mediastinum)**
  - *Superior mediastinal nodes*
    1. Highest mediastinal nodes
    2. Upper paratracheal nodes
    3. Pretracheal and retrotracheal nodes
    4. Lower paratracheal nodes (including azygos nodes)
  - *Aortic nodes*
    5. Subaortic (aortic window)
    6. Para-aortic nodes (ascending aorta or phrenic)
  - *Inferior mediastinal nodes*
    7. Subcarinal nodes
    8. Paraesophageal nodes (below the carina)
    9. Pulmonary ligament nodes
- **N1 nodes (nodes lying distal to the mediastinal pleural reflection)**
    10. Hilar nodes
    11. Interlobar nodes
    12. Lobar nodes
    13. Segmental nodes

In 1983 the ATS created a Committee on Lung Cancer in order to draw up a "map" of regional lymph nodes meeting the requirements of all medical specialties concerned with lung cancer [32]. The guidelines for the development of the classification were: avoid using the terms "mediastinal" and "hilar" since they are not specific from the anatomicoclinical viewpoint; use the relationships with the main anatomical structures identifiable by mediastinoscopy (hence, on the right side: innominate artery, trachea, azygos vein, right main bronchus, origin of the right superior lobe bronchus, carina; on the left side: aorta, left pulmonary artery, ligamentum arteriosum, left main bronchus); and favor the margins that can be visualized on a standard chest X-ray or CT scan.

The following definitions of regional lymph node stations for prethoracotomy staging were proposed:

X. **Supraclavicular nodes**.

2R. **Right upper paratracheal (suprainnominate) nodes**. Nodes to the right of the midline of the trachea between the intersection of the caudal margin of the innominate artery with the trachea and the apex of the lung. Highest right mediastinal nodes are included in this station.

2L. **Left upper paratracheal (supra-aortic) nodes**. Nodes to the left of the midline of the trachea between the upper margin of the aortic arch and the apex of the lung. Highest left mediastinal nodes are included in this station.

4R. **Right lower paratracheal nodes**. Nodes to the right of the midline of the trachea between the cephalic margin of the azygos vein and the intersection of the caudal margin of the brachiocephalic artery with the right side of the trachea. Some pretracheal and paracaval nodes are included in this station.

4L. **Left lower paratracheal nodes**. Nodes to the left of the midline of the trachea between the upper margin of the aortic arch and the level of the carina, medial to the ligamentum arteriosum. Some pretracheal nodes are included in this station.

5. **Aortopulmonary nodes**. Subaortic and para-aortic nodes, lateral to the ligamentum arteriosum or the aorta or left pulmonary artery, proximal to the first branch of the left pulmonary artery.

6. **Anterior mediastinal nodes**. Nodes anterior to the ascending aorta or the innominate artery. Some pretracheal and preaortic nodes are included.

7. **Subcarinal nodes**. Nodes situated caudal to the tracheal carina but not associated with the inferior lobe bronchus or the arteries within the lung.

8. **Paraesophageal nodes**. Nodes dorsal to the posterior wall of the trachea and to the right or left of the esophageal midline. Retrotracheal but not subcarinal nodes are included.

9. **Right or left pulmonary ligament nodes**. Nodes within the right or left pulmonary ligament.

10R. **Right tracheobronchial nodes**. Nodes to the right of the tracheal midline from the level of the cephalic margin of the azygos vein to the origin of the right superior lobe bronchus.

10L. **Left peribronchial nodes**. Nodes to the left of the tracheal midline between the carina and the left superior lobe bronchus, medial to the ligamentum arteriosum.

11. **Intrapulmonary nodes**. Nodes removed in the right or left lung specimen plus those distal to the main bronchus. Interlobar, lobar, and segmental nodes are included. In post-thoracotomy staging they may be subdivided into stations 11, 12, and 13, according to the AJCC classification.

In practice, the revisions to the AJCC classifications were as follows:

– Stations 1, 2, 3, 5, 6, 7, 8, and 9 of the AJCC classifications have remained largely unchanged, but some have been renamed to adhere to the established guidelines.
– The pleural reflection is not taken as reference in the ATS classification because it is deemed not fixed and not radiologically identifiable.
– The use of fixed anatomical landmarks is very helpful to distinguish lymph nodes in critical areas such as stations 4 and 10 (for example, 4R and 10R are separated by the azygos vein, while 4L and 10L are separated by the level of the carina).

A comparison between the two classifications is provided in Table 2.2 [32].

Ten years after these classifications were present-

Table 2.2 – Comparison between AJCC and ATS classifications

Nodal station	AJCC classification	ATS classification
1	Highest mediastinal nodes	Included in station 2
2	Upper paratracheal nodes	Basically unchanged
3	Pretracheal and retrotracheal nodes	If pretracheal, included in stations 2, 4, or 6 depending on anatomical location; if retrotracheal, they are included in station 8
4	Lower paratracheal nodes	The boundaries of this "critical" station are defined
5	Subaortic nodes	Called aortopulmonary to include the lymph nodes along the lateral aspect of the aorta and the main or left pulmonary artery and the nodes of the aortopulmonary window
6	Para-aortic nodes	Called anterior mediastinal nodes; they include some pretracheal and preaortic nodes
7	Subcarinal nodes	Unchanged
8	Paraesophageal nodes	Unchanged
9	Pulmonary ligament nodes	Unchanged
10	Hilar nodes	Called peribronchial on the left side and tracheobronchial on the right side
11	Interlobar nodes	Classified as intrapulmonary
12	Lobar nodes	Included in station 11
13	Segmental nodes	Included in station 11

ed, the two systems were unified in the modified classification of Naruke/ATS–LCSG. This classification was adopted by the AJCC and by the UICC in 1996.

In 1997 Mountain and Dresler [39, 40] published the final version, which provides the anatomical boundaries of the lymph node stations (Fig. 2.2). This classification has had the merit of harmonizing the language of surgeons and pathologists in describing the locoregional spread of lung cancer.

The Mountain/Dresler unified classification includes 14 lymph node stations, identified by name and number (Table 2.3). The lymph node stations considered are those contained within the mediastinal pleural reflection (called N2) and the hilar and intrapulmonary lymph nodes (called N1). N2 nodes include three groups: superior mediastinal nodes (1–4), aortic nodes (5, 6), and inferior mediastinal nodes (7–9). The stations are bilateral (left and right) apart from the highest mediastinal, prevascular and retrotracheal, para-aortic, subcarinal, and paraesophageal nodes.

In addition to the classifications illustrated above, other classifications have been developed by scientific societies [41, 42] or groups of physicians [43]. Among these, the classification of the Japanese Society for Esophageal Disease [41] has become quite well known.

105. **Upper thoracic paraesophageal nodes**. Lateral to the upper thoracic esophagus, between the upper margin of the sternum and the tracheal bifurcation.
106. **Thoracic paratracheal nodes**. Lateral to the thoracic trachea.
107. **Bifurcation nodes**. Anterior to the esophagus, caudal to the tracheal bifurcation, and down to the level of bifurcation of the main bronchi.
108. **Middle thoracic paraesophageal nodes**. Lateral and anterior to the middle thoracic esophagus (proximal portion between the

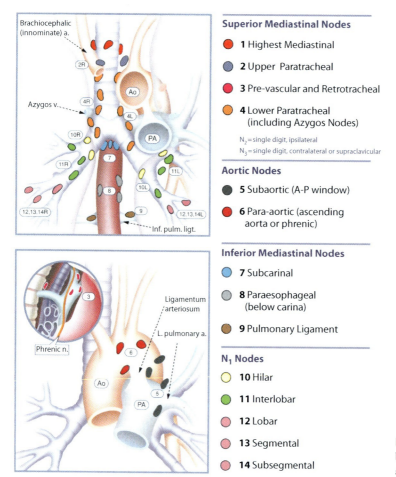

FIG. 2.2 AJCC/UICC classification by Mountain and Dresler. Mountain CF and Dresler CM (1997) [40]

tracheal bifurcation and the esophagogastric junction).
109. **Pulmonary hilar nodes**. In the pulmonary hila around the vessels and main bronchi, after their bifurcation.
110. **Lower thoracic paraesophageal nodes**. Lateral and anterior to the lower thoracic esophagus (distal portion between the tracheal bifurcation and the esophagogastric junction).
111. **Diaphragmatic lymph nodes**. Located around the esophageal hiatus for 5 cm.
112. **Posterior mediastinal nodes**. Posterior to the esophagus, around the thoracic artery.

This classification was modified and supplemented in 1990 by Akiyama [44] who proposed the subdivision of esophageal lymph nodes into seven groups:
1. **Cervical lymph nodes**
    - Deep lateral nodes (spinal accessory nerve chain or level VB)
    - Deep external nodes (or level IV, lateral to the internal jugular vein, including inferiorly the supraclavicular nodes)
    - Deep internal nodes (or level VI, medial to the jugular vein)
2. **Superior mediastinal nodes**
    - Recurrent laryngeal nerve lymphatic chain

Lymph Node Classification

Table 2.3 – AJCC/UICC classification by Mountain and Dresler

Nodal station		Description
Superior mediastinal nodes		
1	Highest mediastinal nodes	Nodes lying above a horizontal line at the upper rim of the brachiocephalic (left innominate) vein where it ascends to the left, crossing in front of the trachea at its midline
2	Upper paratracheal nodes	Nodes lying above a horizontal line drawn tangential to the upper margin of the aortic arch and below the inferior margin of no. 1 nodes
3	Prevascular and retrotracheal nodes	May be designated 3A and 3P
4	Lower paratracheal nodes	**Nodes on the right:** Located to the right of the midline of the trachea between a horizontal line drawn tangential to the upper margin of the aortic arch and a line extending across the right main bronchus at the upper margin of the upper lobe bronchus **Nodes on the left:** Lie to the left of the midline of the trachea between a horizontal line drawn tangential to the upper margin of the aortic arch and a line extending across the left main bronchus at the level of the upper margin of the left upper lobe bronchus They are both contained within the mediastinal pleura. For study purposes lower paratracheal nodes can be divided into superior (4s) and inferior (4i). No. 4s nodes are defined by a horizontal line extending across the trachea and drawn tangential to the cephalic margin of the azygos vein. No. 4i nodes are defined by the lower margin of no. 4s and the caudal margin of no. 4
Aortic nodes		
5	Subaortic nodes (aortopulmonary window)	Subaortic nodes are lateral to the ligamentum arteriosum or the aorta or left pulmonary artery and proximal to the first branch of the left pulmonary artery and lie within the mediastinal pleural envelope
6	Para-aortic nodes (ascending aorta or phrenic)	Nodes lying anterior and lateral to the ascending aorta and the aortic arch or the innominate artery, caudal to a line tangential to the aortic arch
Inferior mediastinal nodes		
7	Subcarinal nodes	Nodes lying caudal to the tracheal carina, but not associated with the lower lobe bronchi or arteries within the lung
8	Paraesophageal nodes (below the carina)	Nodes lying adjacent to the esophageal wall and to the right or left of the midline, excluding subcarinal nodes
9	Pulmonary ligament nodes	Nodes lying within the pulmonary ligament, including those in the posterior wall and lower inferior pulmonary vein
N1 nodes		
10	Hilar nodes	The proximal lobar nodes, distal to the mediastinal pleural reflection and the nodes adjacent to the bronchus intermedius on the right
11	Interlobar nodes	Nodes lying between the lobar bronchi
12	Lobar nodes	Nodes adjacent to the distal lobar bronchi
13	Segmental nodes	Nodes adjacent to the segmental bronchi
14	Subsegmental nodes	Nodes adjacent to the subsegmental bronchi

Source: Mountain CF and Dresler CM (1997) [40]

- Paratracheal nodes
- Nodes of brachiocephalic trunk
- Paraesophageal nodes
- Nodes of infra-aortic arch

3. **Middle mediastinal nodes**
   - Nodes of tracheal bifurcation
   - Pulmonary hilar nodes
   - Paraesophageal nodes

4. **Lower mediastinal nodes**
   - Paraesophageal nodes
   - Diaphragmatic nodes

5. **Superior gastric lymph nodes**
   - Paracardiac nodes
   - Nodes of lesser curvature
   - Nodes of left gastric artery

6. **Celiac trunk nodes**

7. **Common hepatic artery nodes**

To help characterize the nodes of the esophageal region, the Radiation Therapy Oncology Group (RTOG) proposed a classification [45] simply adding new lymph node stations to the already known ones for lung cancer staging (Table 2.4).

Table 2.4 – RTOG classification of lymph nodes draining esophageal cancer

Station	Description
1	Supraclavicular nodes
2R	Right upper paratracheal nodes
2L	Left upper paratracheal nodes
3P	Posterior mediastinal nodes
4R	Right lower paratracheal nodes
4L	Left lower paratracheal nodes
5	Aortopulmonary nodes
6	Anterior mediastinal nodes
7	Subcarinal nodes
8M	Middle paraesophageal nodes
8L	Lower paraesophageal nodes
9	Pulmonary ligament nodes
10R	Right tracheobronchial nodes
10L	Left tracheobronchial nodes
15	Diaphragmatic nodes
16	Paracardiac nodes
17	Left gastric artery nodes
18	Common hepatic artery nodes
19	Splenic artery nodes
20	Celiac nodes

2.3 Upper Abdominal Region

The first detailed description of upper abdominal region nodes was provided by Rouvière [3].

In 1962 the Japanese Research Society for Gastric Cancer (JRSGC) published in Japanese the *General Rules for Gastric Cancer Study*, which were used by surgeons and oncologists for about 30 years with several new editions. The first English edition [46] was published in 1995 and was based on the 12th Japanese edition of the General Rules [47].

These publications introduced a classification of the lymph node stations draining the stomach. These lymph nodes are numbered from 1 to 16 and are classified into four groups according to the location of the primary cancer site. Definition of these groups derived from the results of studies on lymphatic spread patterns from different primary cancer sites, and analysis of survival with respect to the involvement of the various lymph node stations.

In 1998 the JRSGC was transformed into the Japanese Gastric Cancer Association (JGCA) and the 13th edition of the General Rules [48] was published, together with the second English edition of the JGCA classification [49]. Both publications introduced changes in gastric cancer staging, specifically as regards pathological staging and lymph node dissection [50]. The previous four-group classification system was replaced by a system including three groups distinguished in accordance with the gastric site of the primary cancer; a more accurate definition of lymph node groups 11 and 12 was provided; and a new lymph node dissection classification was proposed based on the lymph node groups removed (D0-D1-D2-D3).

Lymph node stations according to the Japanese classification are shown in Fig. 2.3 and listed in Table 2.5, while their subdivision into three groups is shown in Table 2.6.

Also for pancreatic, biliary, and hepatic regions, lymph node classifications have been published by the respective Japanese societies (the Japan Pancreas Society [51], the Liver Cancer Study Group of Japan [52], and the Japanese Society of Biliary Surgery) and the associated staging systems for tumors of the pancreas, of the hepatic and extrahepatic biliary tracts, and of the liver have been subsequently modified [53–56].

For instance, the Japan Pancreas Society published the first English edition of the *Classification of Pancreatic Carcinoma* in 1996 [56]. This edition was based on the fourth Japanese edition of the *General*

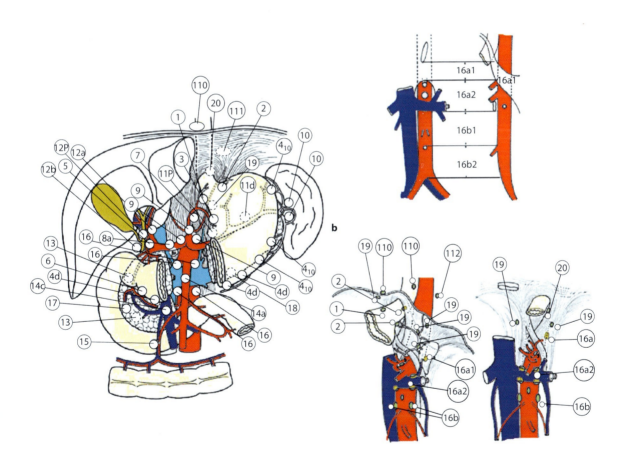

FIG. 2.3 a,b Illustration of the classification of regional lymph nodes of the stomach according to the Japanese Gastric Cancer Association. **a** Anterior view with cross-section of stomach and pancreas. **b** Detail of the location of the lymph nodes around the abdominal aorta. **c** Detail of the location of lymph nodes in the esophageal hiatus of the diaphragm, of the infradiaphragmatic nodes and para-aortic nodes. Japanese Gastric Cancer Association (1998) [49]

Table 2.5 – Classification of regional lymph nodes of the stomach according to the Japanese Gastric Cancer Association (JGCA)

	Name	Description
1	Right paracardial nodes	Located at the level of the esophagogastric junction, along the branch of the left gastric artery
2	Left paracardial nodes	Located to the left of the cardia. They also include the lymph nodes around the cardioesophageal branches of the inferior diaphragmatic artery
3	Nodes along the lesser gastric curvature	On the lesser curvature of the stomach, along the lower branch of the left gastric artery
4	Nodes along the greater gastric curvature	Located around the gastroepiploic arteries, they are therefore located close to the greater curvature of the stomach; they are subdivided, based on blood flow, into right-side nodes (**4d nodes along the right gastroepiploic vessels**), around the right epiploic artery beyond the level of the first collateral leading to the stomach, and left-side nodes (4s). The left-side nodes are further subdivided into proximal (**4sa nodes along the short gastric vessels**), located at the level of the short vessels, and distal (**4sb nodes along the left gastroepiploic vessels**), located along the left gastroepiploic artery
5	Suprapyloric nodes	Located around the right gastric artery and close to the upper pylorus, downward lymph nodes 3
6	Subpyloric nodes	Located at the level of the lower pylorus and around the right gastroepiploic artery, from its point of origin to the origin of the lateral branch heading toward the greater gastric curvature
7	Nodes along the left gastric artery	Located at the level of the left gastric artery, between its origin from the celiac trunk and its left end at the level of the stomach, where it divides into its two terminal branches
8	Nodes along the common hepatic artery	Located along the common hepatic artery, from its point of origin to the hepatic artery, at the point of origin of the gastroduodenal artery; they are subdivided into: – **8a anterosuperior group** – **8p posterior group**
9	Nodes around the celiac artery	Located around the celiac trunk; they include the lymph nodes around the origins of the hepatic artery and splenic artery
10	Nodes at the splenic hilum	Located at the level of the splenic hilum, beyond the tail of the pancreas; they are separated from lymph nodes 4sb through the first gastric collateral of the gastroepiploic artery
11	Nodes along the splenic artery	They include the lymph nodes located along the splenic artery, the celiac trunk, and the final portion of the tail of pancreas; they are subdivided into: – **11p proximal** – **11d distal**
12	Nodes of hepatoduodenal ligament	They are divided into three subgroups: – **12a along the hepatic artery**, located at the level of the upper left of the hepatic pedicle and of the hepatic artery proper – **12b along the bile duct**, on the right side of the common hepatic artery and the lower common bile duct – **12p behind the portal vein**, located posterior to the portal vein
13	Posterior pancreaticoduodenal nodes	Located on the posterior aspect of the head of the pancreas
14a	Nodes along the superior mesenteric artery	Located along the superior mesenteric artery, at the root of the mesentery
14v	Nodes along the superior mesenteric vein	Located along the superior mesenteric vein, at the root of the mesentery
15	Nodes along the middle colic vessels	Located around the middle colic artery

Table 2.5 – (*continued*) Classification of regional lymph nodes of the stomach according to the Japanese Gastric Cancer Association (JGCA)

Name		Description
16a1	Nodes of the aortic hiatus	They include the lymph nodes around the abdominal aorta; they are bordered laterally by the corresponding renal hila
16a2	Nodes around the abdominal aorta (from the upper margin of the celiac trunk to the lower margin of the left renal vein)	
16b1	Nodes around the abdominal aorta (from the lower margin of the left renal vein to the upper margin of the inferior mesenteric artery)	
16b2	Nodes around the abdominal aorta (from the upper margin of the inferior mesenteric artery to the aortic bifurcation)	
17	Nodes on the anterior aspect of the pancreatic head	Located on to the anterior aspect of the head of the pancreas
18	Nodes along the inferior margin of the pancreas	Located along the inferior margin of the pancreas
19	Infradiaphragmatic nodes	Located below the diaphragm
20	Nodes of the esophageal hiatus of the diaphragm	Included in the Japanese stomach tumor classification when invasion of the esophagus occurs
110	Paraesophageal nodes of the lower chest	
111	Supradiaphragmatic nodes	
112	Posterior mediastinal nodes	

Table 2.6 – Groupings of the regional lymph nodes of the stomach (groups 1–3) according to the Japanese Gastric Cancer Association

Lymph nodes		Location					
		LMU/MUL MLU/UML	LD/L	LM/M/ML	MU/UM	U	E+
1	Right paracardial nodes	1	2	1	1	1	
2	Left paracardial nodes	1	Met	3	1	1	
3	Nodes along the lesser curvature	1	1	1	1	1	
4sa	Nodes along the short gastric vessels	1	Met	3	1	1	
4sb	Nodes along the left gastroepiploic vessels	1	3	1	1	1	
4d	Nodes along the right gastroepiploic vessels	1	1	1	1	2	
5	Suprapyloric nodes	1	1	1	1	3	
6	Infrapyloric nodes	1	1	1	1	3	
7	Nodes along the left gastric artery	2	2	2	2	2	

Met: lymph nodes regarded as distant metastasis,
E+: lymph node stations reclassified in case of esophageal invasion,
U, M, L, D: indicate the different parts of the stomach (*U* upper third, *M* middle third, *L* lower third) and invasion sites (*D* duodenum). If more than one side of the stomach is involved, the different sides must be listed by decreasing degree of involvement, with the first letter indicating the side in which the bulky tumor is located

Source: Japanese Gastric Cancer Association (1998) [49]

Table 2.6 – (continued) Groupings of the regional lymph nodes of the stomach (groups 1–3) according to the Japanese Gastric Cancer Association

Lymph nodes		Location					
		LMU/MUL MLU/UML	LD/L	LM/M/ML	MU/UM	U	E+
8a	Nodes along the common hepatic artery (anterosuperior group)	2	2	2	2	2	
8b	Nodes along the common hepatic artery (posterior group)	3	3	3	3	3	
9	Nodes around the celiac artery	2	2	2	2	2	
10	Nodes at the splenic hilum	2	Met	3	2	2	
11p	Nodes along the proximal splenic artery	2	2	2	2	2	
11d	Nodes along the distal splenic artery	2	Met	3	2	2	
12a	Nodes of the hepatoduodenal ligament (along the hepatic artery)	2	2	2	2	3	
12b	Nodes of the hepatoduodenal ligament (along the bile duct)	3	3	3	3	3	
12p	Nodes of the hepatoduodenal ligament (behind the portal vein)	3	3	3	3	3	
13	Nodes on the posterior aspect of the pancreatic head	3	3	3	Met	Met	
14a	Nodes along the superior mesenteric artery	Met	Met	Met	Met	Met	
14v	Nodes along the superior mesenteric vein	2	2	3	3	Met	
15	Nodes along the middle colic vessels	Met	Met	Met	Met	Met	
16a1	Nodes of the aortic hiatus	Met	Met	Met	Met	Met	
16a2	Nodes around the abdominal aorta (from the upper margin of the celiac trunk to the lower margin of the left renal vein)	3	3	3	3	3	
16b1	Nodes around the abdominal aorta (from the lower margin of the left renal vein to the upper margin of the inferior mesenteric artery)	3	3	3	3	3	
16b2	Nodes around the abdominal aorta (from the upper margin of the inferior mesenteric artery to the aortic bifurcation)	Met	Met	Met	Met	Met	
17	Nodes on the anterior aspect of the pancreatic head	Met	Met	Met	Met	Met	
18	Nodes along the inferior margin of the pancreas	Met	Met	Met	Met	Met	
19	Infradiaphragmatic nodes	3	Met	Met	3	3	2
20	Nodes in the esophageal hiatus of the diaphragm	3	Met	Met	3	3	1
110	Paraesophageal nodes in the lower chest	Met	Met	Met	Met	Met	3
111	Supradiaphragmatic nodes	Met	Met	Met	Met	Met	3
112	Posterior mediastinal nodes	Met	Met	Met	Met	Met	3

Met: lymph nodes regarded as distant metastasis,
E+: lymph node stations reclassified in case of esophageal invasion,
U, M, L, D: indicate the different parts of the stomach (*U* upper third, *M* middle third, *L* lower third) and invasion sites (*D* duodenum). If more than one side of the stomach is involved, the different sides must be listed by decreasing degree of involvement, with the first letter indicating the side in which the bulky tumor is located

Source: Japanese Gastric Cancer Association (1998) [49]

Rules for the Study of Pancreatic Cancer published in 1993 [55] (the previous Japanese editions had been published in 1980 [51], 1982 [53], and 1986 [54]). In 1997, the Review Committee of the General Rules for the Study of Pancreatic Cancer made a comparison between the Japanese classification and the fifth edition of the UICC classification [57]. On this basis, it started preparing the fifth edition of the General Rules, taking into consideration the limitations and advantages of both classifications. Unfortunately, when in 2002 the fifth edition of the General Rules was published, at the same time the sixth edition of the UICC classification was released, and it was not possible to include in the new General Rules [58, 59] the changes introduced in the latest edition of the UICC classification.

The classifications proposed do not differ as to the nomenclature and numbering from the classification of lymph node stations of the stomach, which we have therefore taken as reference for the entire upper abdominal region. For instance, the classification of the main lymph node stations draining the pancreas includes lymph nodes already listed for gastric cancer from 5 to 18 (Fig. 2.4) [60, 61]. The only difference is that some lymph node groups are further subdivided, specifically:

- **Lymph nodes 12** (nodes of the hepatoduodenal ligament) are further subdivided into:
  - 12a1 and 12a2, 12b1 and 12b2, 12p1 and 12p2 (where numbers 1 and 2 differentiate the lymph nodes into superior and inferior groups, respectively)
- **Lymph nodes 13** (posterior pancreaticoduodenal) are further subdivided into:
  - 13a (superior group) and 13b (inferior group)
- **Lymph nodes 14** (nodes along the superior mesenteric artery) are further subdivided into:
  - 14a: Nodes at the origin of the superior mesenteric artery
  - 14b: Nodes at the origin of the inferior pancreaticoduodenal artery
  - 14c: Nodes at the origin of the middle colic artery
  - 14d: Nodes at the origin of the jejunal arteries
- **Lymph nodes 17** (anterior pancreaticoduodenal) are further subdivided into:
  - 17a (superior group) and 17b (inferior group)

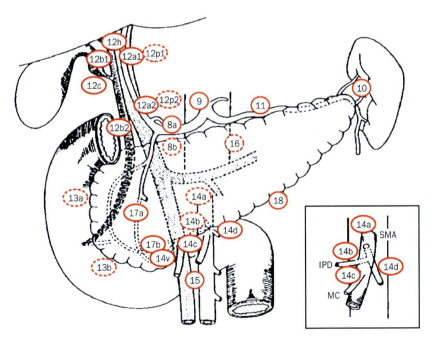

FIG. 2.4 Main lymph node stations draining the pancreas. *SMA* superior mesenteric artery, *IPD* inferior pancreatoduodenal artery, *MC* middle colic artery, *J* jejunal artery. Adapted from Pedrazzoli S, Beger HG, Obertop H et al. (1999) [61]

2.4 Pelvic Region

As mentioned by Gregoire [6], lymph drainage of the pelvis has been described in anatomy and surgery textbooks but, unlike other anatomical regions, such as the head and neck and mediastinum regions, there is no universally accepted classification. The lack of a standard nomenclature largely derives from the technical difficulties involved in the identification, surgical dissection, and anatomicopathological evaluation of pelvic lymph nodes. For instance, the nodes located along the pelvic walls are continuously connected to the internal and external iliac vessels and therefore cannot be characterized distinctly. Moreover, the surgical field is narrow, making it difficult to evaluate the anatomical boundaries of individual lymph node stations; detailed pathological examination of these lymph nodes is moreover altered by infiltrating fatty and fibrous tissue and by inflammation.

As for the lymph nodes draining the female genitalia, after the initial description of the lymphatic system made by Reiffenstuhl [62] in 1964 and Plentl and Friedman [63] in 1971, an attempt to establish a classification of the lymph nodes of interest to gynecological oncology was made by Mangan et al. [64]. These authors proposed a system including nine major lymph node groups:

- Group 1. Para-aortic lymph nodes
- Group 2. Common iliac lymph nodes

Table 2.7 – Subdivision of paraaortic and pelvic lymph nodes

Type	Description
Para-aortic lymph nodes	
Paracaval nodes	Located to the right of the vena cava
Precaval nodes	Located anterior to the vena cava
Postcaval nodes	Located posterior to the vena cava when the vein is mobilized to the left
Deep intercavoaortic nodes	To the right of the aorta, between the aorta and the vena cava, above the lumbar vessels
Superficial intercavoaortic nodes	To the right of the aorta, between the aorta and the vena cava, below the lumbar vessels
Preaortic nodes	Anterior to the aorta
Para-aortic nodes	Lateral to the aorta
Postaortic nodes	Posterior to the aorta
Pelvic lymph nodes	
Common iliac nodes	Around the common iliac vessels
– Medial subgroup	
– Superficial lateral subgroup	
– Deep lateral subgroup	In a space delimited laterally by the psoas muscle, medially by the common iliac vein and by the two iliolumbar veins, and posteriorly by the ischiatic nerve and by the origin of the obturator nerve
External iliac nodes	
Internal iliac nodes	
Deep obturator nodes	
Superficial obturator nodes	
Presacral nodes	
Parametrial nodes	

- Groups 3 and 4. External iliac lymph nodes
- Group 5. Obturator lymph nodes
- Group 6. Inferior gluteal lymph nodes
- Group 7. Hypogastric lymph nodes (internal iliac)
- Groups 8 and 9. Presacral lymph nodes

While these studies played a key role for the understanding of the lymphatic pathways of ovarian tumors, this classification was not widely adopted. In 1992 a study was published on pelvic and para-aortic lymph node dissection in patients affected by gynecological tumors, in order to evaluate the number of nodes present in each lymph node group and review existing nomenclature [65]. This study divided para-aortic nodes into eight groups and pelvic nodes into seven groups (Table 2.7).

We agree with Gregoire [6] in believing that the pelvic lymph node classification most suitable for radiotherapy planning is the one that associates lymph node groups with the distribution of the main arteries. For this classification, see Chapter 1.

Anatomicoradiological Boundaries 3

With the introduction in clinical practice of new radiological imaging techniques such as computed tomography (CT) and magnetic resonance imaging (MRI) the need was felt to transfer onto CT scans the anatomical boundaries of lymph node stations as described by surgeons.

Computed tomography images are not always able to visualize what the surgeon has described; however, by means of identifiable structures, they provide anatomicoradiological references for the identification of lymph node sites.

Specifically, progress in radiotherapy technology and the introduction of conformational techniques have made it necessary to provide exact definition of the boundaries of anatomical structures which are sites of macroscopic or microscopic tumors. In this regard, a landmark guide is provided by the volume published by Gregoire, Scalliet, and Ang in 2004 [6] which defines the criteria for appropriate definition of clinical target volumes (CTVs) [7, 8] in modern conformal radiotherapy and in intensity modulated radiation therapy (IMRT). In Italy, again in 2004, Valentini et al. developed a software tool called TIGER (Tutorial for Image Guided External Radiotherapy) [66] intended as a contouring training tool and based on the set of images of the Visible Human Project, with the purpose of facilitating the interpretation of CT images and, especially, the contouring of radiotherapy volumes.

Based on our experience, for the four anatomical regions considered, we report the anatomicoradiological boundaries for identifying lymph node structures.

3.1 Head and Neck Region

Definition of the nodal neck levels and related anatomical boundaries described by Robbins were originally proposed for surgical procedures and are not always easily identifiable on CT scans. Adapting the anatomicosurgical boundaries in order to identify CTVs for radiotherapy is neither simple nor easy. Moreover, in radiotherapy the neck is immobilized without rotation of the head, while in surgery the position of the neck can be rotated.

In 1999, a group of authors from the school of Rotterdam [67] addressed the issue of CT-based definition of target volumes for stage N0 of the neck and published an initial transposition of the boundaries of the six surgical levels of the neck on CT scans, based on an anatomical study of human cadavers. In the same year, other authors also published their contributions to this topic, in particular, Som [68, 69], a radiologist and member of the committee of the AHNS for the 1998 revision of the 1991 AAO-HNS classification. Som attempted to introduce boundaries for the nodal levels of the Robbins classification that would be easily visible in radiological imaging (CT and MRI), in order to provide a system which, being consistent with that established in the previous literature, could unify anatomical imaging criteria with the AJCC and AAO-HNS nodal classifications and clarify some uncertainties.

In the same period, several atlases of cross-sectional radiological anatomy of head and neck nodes were published; however, these failed to define the boundaries of the various nodal regions [70–72].

In 2000, Gregoire [26] published guidelines for the selection and delineation of lymph node target volumes in head and neck tumor patients, and provided recommendations for nodal station contouring in that region. He used the surgical classification in levels (adding retropharyngeal lymph nodes), but converting the anatomical boundaries into radiological boundaries, which can be identified more easily on CT or MRI than those of the surgical field. These recommendations are based on the radiological classification proposed by Som et al. [68] and modified by Robbins [21] and agree fairly well with those proposed by Nowak [67].

The studies of Nowak and Levendag (Rotterdam) and Gregoire (Brussels), were followed by further studies which added the anatomical margins of the nodal levels of the neck on CT scans [73, 74]. In Italy the Lombardia Cooperative Group of the Italian Society of Radiation Oncology (*Associazione Italiana di Radioterapia Oncologica*, AIRO) proposed guidelines for delineation of head and neck nodes on axial CT images [75, 76].

The contouring guidelines of the schools of Brussels and Rotterdam were the most commonly used in radiotherapy, but presented some differences in terms of boundaries and sizes; consequently, the need was felt to unify terminology and recommendations for contouring the individual nodal stations. The main differences between the two systems concerned the definition of the cranial edge of levels II and V, the posterior edge of levels II, III, IV, and V, and the caudal edge of level VI.

Thus, the two groups have resolved the differences between their respective contouring guidelines [77]. An interdisciplinary working group was created, including members from both the original Brussels and Rotterdam groups. At the end of 2003, the group published its "consensus guidelines" which have been endorsed by the major European and American scientific societies (RTOG, EORTC, GO-ERTEC, NCIC, and DAHANCA) (Table 3.1) [78].

The radiological boundaries for delineation of nodal levels have been validated surgically, and a correspondence was observed between radiological and surgical boundaries, except for the posterior edge of level IIa (whose surgical edge is defined by the spinal accessory nerve, while the radiological edge is defined by the internal jugular vein) [79].

Based on the validation of these guidelines, for nodal neck contouring, we adopted the radiological boundaries of the "consensus guidelines" (Table 3.1).

3.2 Mediastinal Region

Currently, the regional lymph node classification for lung cancer staging, recommended for radiation therapy planning [80], is the 1996 AJCC-UICC classification by Mountain and Dresler [40]. These authors mapped nodal stations describing them with the help of anatomical boundaries and four lines having the function of marking the craniocaudal border of some of the nodal stations classified (Fig. 3.1):

- **Line 1.** Horizontal, at the upper rim of the brachiocephalic (left innominate) vein, where it ascends to the left, crossing in front of the trachea at its midline
- **Line 2.** Horizontal, tangential to the upper edge of the aortic arch
- **Line 3.** Extending across the right main bronchus at the upper edge of the right upper lobe bronchus
- **Line 4.** Extending across the left main bronchus at the upper edge of the left upper lobe bronchus

Anatomicoradiological Boundaries

Table 3.1 – Boundaries of neck node levels according to the 2003 consensus guidelines

Level	Anatomical boundaries					
	Cranial	Caudal	Medial	Lateral	Anterior	Posterior
Ia	Geniohyoid m., plane tangent to basilar edge of mandible	Plane tangent to body of hyoid bone	n.a.[a]	Medial edge of ant. belly of digastric m.	Symphysis menti, platysma m.	Body of hyoid bone[b]
Ib	Mylohyoid m., cranial edge of submandibular gland	Plane through central part of hyoid bone	Lateral edge of ant. belly of digastric m.	Basilar edge/inner side of mandible, platysma m., skin	Symphysis menti, platysma m.	Posterior edge of submandibular gland
IIa	Caudal edge of lateral process of C1	Caudal edge of the body of hyoid bone	Medial edge of int. carotid artery, paraspinal (levator scapulae) m.	Medial edge of sternocleidomastoid m.	Post. edge of submandibular gland; ant. edge of int. carotid artery; post. edge of post. belly of digastric m.	Post. border of int. jugular vein
IIb	Caudal edge of lateral process of C1	Caudal edge of the body of hyoid bone	Medial edge of int. carotid artery, paraspinal (levator scapulae) m.	Medial edge of sternocleidomastoid m.	Post. border of int. jugular vein	Post. border of the sternocleidomastoid m.
III	Caudal edge of the body of hyoid bone	Caudal edge of cricoid cartilage	Int. edge of carotid artery, paraspinal (scalene) m.	Medial edge of sternocleidomastoid m.	Posterolateral edge of the sternohyoid m.; ant. edge of sternocleidomastoid m.	Post. edge of the sternocleidomastoid m.
IV	Caudal edge of cricoid cartilage	2 cm cranial to sternoclavicular joint	Medial edge of int. carotid artery, paraspinal (scalene) m.	Medial edge of sternocleidomastoid m.	Anteromedial edge of sternocleidomastoid m.	Post. edge of the sternocleidomastoid m.
V	Cranial edge of body of hyoid bone	CT slice encompassing the transverse cervical vessels[c]	Paraspinal (levator scapulae, splenius capitis) m.	Platysma m., skin	Post. edge of the sternocleidomastoid m.	Anterolateral border of the trapezius m.
VI	Caudal edge of body of thyroid cartilage[d]	Sternal manubrium	n.a.	Medial edges of thyroid gland, skin and anteromedial edge of sternocleidomastoid m.	Skin; platysma m.	Separation between trachea and esophagus[e]
RP	Base of skull	Cranial edge of the body of hyoid bone	Midline	Medial edge of int. carotid artery	Fascia under the pharyngeal mucosa	Prevertebral m. (longus colli, longus capitis)

[a] Midline structure lying between the medial borders of the anterior bellies of the digastric muscles
[b] The insertion of the thyroid muscle is often interposed between level Ia and the body of the hyoid bone
[c] For NPC, the reader is referred to the original description of the UICC/AJCC 1997 edition of the Ho's triangle. In essence, the fatty planes below and around the clavicle down to the trapezius muscle
[d] For paratracheal and recurrent nodes, the cranial border is the caudal edge of the cricoid cartilage
[e] For pretracheal nodes, trachea and anterior edge of cricoid cartilage

Source: Modified from Gregoire V, Levendag P, Ang KK, et al. (2003) [78]

Subsequently, Cymbalista [81] illustrated Mountain's classification on CT, to help radiologists familiarize themselves with the new classification of the regional lymph nodes involved in lung cancer.

In 1999, an atlas of cross-sectional anatomy was published for the definition of nodal regions, including mediastinal ones [72], and in 2004, Gregoire [6] indicated the anatomical boundaries for contouring four main nodal areas:

1. Parasternal
2. Brachiocephalic
3. Intertracheobronchial
4. Posterior mediastinal

Despite this, Mountain's anatomical definitions of nodal stations are not fully explanatory for individual nodal station contouring in conformal radiotherapy.

In 2003, at the National Congress of the AIRO, Vinciguerra et al. presented a communication on the program for nodal CTV contouring using easily identifiable anatomical boundaries [82].

A similar study was conducted at the University of Michigan by an interdisciplinary working group, which proposed radiological boundaries in order to define on CT cross-sectional images the lymph node stations described by Mountain and Dresler [83].

Table 3.2 illustrates the anatomicoradiological boundaries of mediastinal nodal stations up to station 8 based on our experience. To identify pulmonary ligament nodes (stations 9R and 9L), hilar nodes (stations 10R and 10L), and interlobar nodes (stations 11R and 11L) we have preferred a non-schematic description, provided here below:

- **Pulmonary ligament lymph nodes (stations 9R and 9L)** are paired lymph nodes, left and right, lying within the pulmonary ligaments. The region in which these nodes are located is difficult to identify on CT scan, since the pulmonary ligament itself is not always clearly visible.
- **Hilar lymph nodes (stations 10R and 10L)** are adjacent to the bifurcation of the main bronchus in left and right lobar bronchi. Their upper and lower limits are marked, respectively, by a plane cutting the main bronchi just below the carina and by a plane passing through the caudal limit of the main bronchi. These nodes are frequently located between the right and left pulmonary arteries and between the right and left main bronchi.
- **Interlobar lymph nodes (stations 11R and 11L)** are located in the fatty tissue lying between the lobar bronchi.

The cranial edge of these nodal stations is therefore provided by the appearance of lobar bronchi, while the caudal edge is provided by the further subdivision of the lobe bronchi on the axial plane.

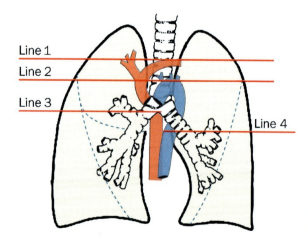

FIG. 3.1 Graphic representation of the four main lines for checking mediastinal node stations

Anatomicoradiological Boundaries

Table 3.2 – Boundaries of the main mediastinal lymph node stations

Station	Anatomical boundaries					
	Cranial	Caudal	Medial	Lateral	Anterior	Posterior
1R	Thoracic inlet[a]	Horizontal plane passing through line 1[b]	Trachea, thyroid	Right lung, right common carotid artery	Right clavicle, right brachiocephalic vein, thyroid	Anterior limit of station 3P, right subclavian artery
1L	Thoracic inlet[a]	Horizontal plane passing through line 1[b]	Trachea, thyroid	Left lung	Left subclavian vein, thyroid, left clavicle, left brachiocephalic vein	Anterior limit of station 3P, left subclavian artery, left common carotid artery
2R	Horizontal plane passing through line 1[b]	Horizontal plane passing through line 2[b]	Trachea, brachiocephalic trunk, station 2L	Right lung, right subclavian artery	Brachiocephalic trunk, right brachiocephalic vein, station 3A	Anterior limit of station 3P, trachea
2L	Horizontal plane passing through line 1[b]	Horizontal plane passing through line 2[b]	Trachea, station 2R	Left subclavian artery, left lung	Brachiocephalic trunk and left brachiocephalic vein	Anterior limit of station 3P, trachea
3A	Horizontal plane tangential to the top of sternal manubrium	Horizontal plane passing through line 2[b]	–	Right brachiocephalic vein, right and left lung	Sternum, clavicles	Thyroid, brachiocephalic trunk, right and left brachiocephalic veins
3P	Thoracic inlet[a]	Horizontal plane passing through carina	Esophagus	Right and left lung, right and left subclavian artery, descending aorta	Trachea, station 1R, station 1L, station 2R, station 2L, station 4R, station 4L	Esophagus, vertebral body
4R	Horizontal plane passing through line 2[b]	Horizontal plane passing through line 3[b]	Aortic arch, trachea, station 4L	Right lung, superior vena cava, arch of the azygos	Right brachiocephalic vein, aortic arch, ascending aorta	Right anterior-lateral wall of trachea, station 3P, right main bronchus
4L	Horizontal plane passing through line 2[b]	Horizontal plane passing through line 4[b]	Trachea, station 4R	Aortic arch, left pulmonary artery, ligamentum arteriosum	Ascending aorta, right and left pulmonary artery	Left anterior-lateral wall of the trachea, descending aorta, station 3P, left main bronchus
5	Horizontal plane passing through inferior border of aortic arch	Horizontal plane passing through the most inferior aspect of left pulmonary artery	Ligamentum arteriosum, ascending aorta, main pulmonary artery	Left lung	Posterior limit of station 6	Descending aorta, left pulmonary artery

[a] The thoracic inlet marks the cervicothoracic junction. It can be represented by an imaginary plane tangential to the first rib and with oblique direction from the top downward and from the back toward the front

[b] For the definitions of the four main lines, see the text

Table 3.2 – (*continued*) Boundaries of the main mediastinal lymph node stations

Station	Anatomical boundaries					
	Cranial	Caudal	Medial	Lateral	Anterior	Posterior
6	Horizontal plane passing through line 2[b]	Horizontal plane passing through auricle of right atrium	–	Right and left lung	Sternum	Superior vena cava, left brachiocephalic vein, aortic arch, ascending aorta, pulmonary trunk, station 5
7	Horizontal plane extending across the carina	Horizontal plane passing through the most inferior aspect of right pulmonary artery (where the two main bronchi are neatly separated)	–	Medial wall of right and left main bronchi and of middle lobe bronchus	Right pulmonary artery	Esophagus, station 8
8	Inferior limit of station 3P	Diaphragm	–	Descending aorta, right lung, azygos vein	Left atrium, esophagus, station 7	Vertebral body

[a] The thoracic inlet marks the cervicothoracic junction. It can be represented by an imaginary plane tangential to the first rib and with oblique direction from the top downward and from the back toward the front
[b] For the definitions of the four main lines, see the text

3.3 Upper Abdominal Region

The experience with CTV contouring of tumors of the upper abdominal region is rather limited.

In 1999, a cross-sectional nodal atlas was published for the definition of nodal regions, including those located in the upper abdominal regions [72].

Gregoire [6] described the different lymphatic drainage areas, and defined three main levels, IA, IIA, and IIIA, for the gastroenteric district:
- **Level IA**, "celiac level," which he defines as located in front of the T12 vertebra
- **Level IIA**, "superior mesenteric level," located at the level of the L1 vertebra
- **Level IIIA**, "inferior mesenteric level," located in front of the L3 vertebra

Recently, some authors [84] have described the correspondence between the lymph node stations draining the stomach, numbered according to the Japanese classification, and the lymph node areas identified by Martinez-Monge [72] on CT images.

Table 3.3 lists the anatomicoradiological boundaries of lymph node stations defined on the basis of our contouring experience and based on the Japanese classification.

3.4 Pelvic Region

In the past, several studies were carried out to evaluate coverage of pelvic lymph node CTVs by radiotherapy using the traditional four-field box technique. Greer et al. [85] suggested some anatomical boundaries for the definition of particular lymph node regions based on intraoperative measurements: with respect to the sacral promontory, the aortic bifurcation is located 6.7 cm cranially; the bifurcation of the right common iliac artery is located

Anatomicoradiological Boundaries

Table 3.3 – Anatomicoradiological boundaries of lymph node stations of the upper abdominal region

Station		Anatomical boundaries					
		Cranial	Caudal	Medial	Lateral	Anterior	Posterior
1	Right paracardial nodes	Plane through upper border of cardia (~T9–T10)	Plane through lower border of cardia (~T10–T11)	Cardia	Liver (superiorly), left diaphragmatic crus (inferiorly)	Liver	Cardia (superiorly), abdominal aorta (inferiorly)
2	Left paracardial nodes	Plane through upper border of cardia (~T9–T10)	Plane through lower border of cardia (~T10–T11)	Cardia	Stomach	Liver	Cardia (superiorly), abdominal aorta (inferiorly)
3	Nodes along the lesser curvature[a]	Plane through upper limit of the body and fundus of the stomach	Plane through lower limit of the body and fundus of the stomach	Left lobe of liver	Lesser gastric curvature	Fatty tissue	Stomach
7	Nodes along the left gastric artery						
4	Nodes along the greater gastric curvature	Plane through upper limit of the body and fundus of the stomach	Plane through lower limit of body of stomach	Greater gastric curvature	Intestine and left colic (splenic) flexure	Intestine	Spleen, anterior limit of station 10
5	Suprapyloric nodes	Plane through superior border of the pyloric region of the stomach	Plane through lower limit of the hepatic hilum	Fatty tissue	Ascending colon or liver (near the bed of the gallbladder)	Intestine	Pylorus
6	Infrapyloric nodes	Plane through upper limit of duodenum	1–1.5 cm caudal to the pylorus	Fatty tissue	Right colic (hepatic) flexure of the ascending colon or liver (near the bed of the gallbladder)	Intestine	Duodenum
8	Nodes along the common hepatic artery	Horizontal plane through the origin of celiac trunk	Intervertebral space T11–T12	Celiac trunk region (superiorly), pancreas (inferiorly)	Liver	Left lobe of liver (superiorly), antropyloric region (inferiorly)	Inferior vena cava
12	Nodes in the hepatoduodenal ligament						
9	Nodes around the celiac artery	Horizontal plane through the origin of celiac trunk	Plane passing above the origin of the mesenteric vessels	–	Liver (to the right), stomach (to the left)	Stomach	Aorta

[a] Station 19 (infradiaphragmatic lymph nodes) has been considered together with station 3 (lymph nodes along the lesser curvature)
[b] Station 15 (nodes along the middle colic vessels) has been considered together with station 14 (nodes along the superior mesenteric vessels)

Table 3.3 – (*continued*) Anatomicoradiological boundaries of lymph node stations of the upper abdominal region

Station		Anatomical boundaries					
		Cranial	Caudal	Medial	Lateral	Anterior	Posterior
10	Nodes at the splenic hilum	Superior limit of the vessels of splenic hilum	Lower limit of the vessels of splenic hilum	Body of stomach (superiorly), tail of pancreas (inferiorly)	Spleen	Posterior limit of station 4	Spleen
11	Nodes along the splenic artery	Superior limit of splenic artery	Lower limit of splenic artery	Abdominal aorta	Fatty tissue	Body of pancreas	Splenic hilum
13	Posterior pancreaticoduodenal nodes	Plane through superior border of the head of pancreas	Plane through lower border of the head of pancreas	Abdominal aorta	Descending (2nd) part of duodenum	Head of pancreas	Inferior vena cava
14	Nodes along the superior mesenteric vessels[b]	Superior limit of mesenteric vessels (~interspace T11–T12)	Plane through the origin of the superior mesenteric artery (~T12)	–	Head of pancreas	Head and isthmus of the pancreas	Abdominal aorta
16	Nodes around the abdominal aorta	Plane through upper limit of the celiac trunk	Aortic division into iliac vessels	–	–	–	Vertebral bodies
17	Anterior pancreaticoduodenal nodes	Plane through superior border of the head of pancreas	Plane through lower border of the head of pancreas	Intestine	Superior (1st) and descending (2nd) part of duodenum	Intestine	Head of pancreas
18	Nodes along the inferior margin of the pancreas	Plane through superior border of the body of pancreas	Caudal limit of the body and tail of pancreas	–	–	Head and tail of pancreas	Abdominal aorta, left kidney, and left suprarenal gland
20	Nodes in the esophageal hiatus of the diaphragm	Carina	Esophageal hiatus of the diaphragm	–	Right: lung (superiorly), inferior vena cava (inferiorly) Left: left pulmonary hilum (superiorly), thoracic and abdominal aorta (inferiorly)	Bronchi (superiorly), heart and liver (inferiorly)	Vertebral bodies
110	Paraesophageal nodes in the lower thorax						
111	Supradiaphragmatic nodes						
112	Posterior mediastinal nodes						

[a] Station 19 (infradiaphragmatic lymph nodes) has been considered together with station 3 (lymph nodes along the lesser curvature)
[b] Station 15 (nodes along the middle colic vessels) has been considered together with station 14 (nodes along the superior mesenteric vessels)

1.7 cm cranially; and the bifurcation of the left common iliac artery is located 1.4 cm cranially. Bonin et al. [86] using lymphangiography in patients with cancer of the uterine cervix, evaluated the mean distance between the position of pelvic lymph nodes and some landmarks on the pelvic bones.

Zunino et al. [87] also evaluated adequacy of CTV coverage in carcinoma of the uterine cervix obtained by the traditional box technique and, by means of an anatomical study on human cadavers, identified the aortic bifurcation and the position of the pelvic lymph nodes. These authors observed that the bifurcation of the aorta is located 3.5 cm (in 5% of cases), 4 cm (20%), or 2.5 cm (15%) from the sacral promontory and that it is located at the level of the inferior edge of the L4 vertebra in 80% of cases.

The Martinez-Monge cross-sectional nodal atlas illustrates location of the pelvic lymph node regions [72] without providing explicit definition of the boundaries of the various nodal regions.

In order to define pelvic lymph node stations on CT scans, various authors have proposed guidelines taking vascular structures as points of reference. For instance, Roeske et al. [88] suggested contrast-enhanced pelvic vessels plus a 2-cm margin to ensure coverage of the pelvic lymph nodes at risk or not directly visible on CT scans. Nutting et al. [89], on the other hand, defined pelvic lymph node CTV in patients with negative nodes by adding a 1-cm margin around the internal, external, and common iliac vessels.

Chao and Lin [90], to assist radiation oncologists in correct lymph node target delineation, carried out a study to determine the spatial orientation of para-aortic, pelvic, and inguinal lymph nodes on the basis of their relationship with the adjacent vascular structures, using lymphangiography on CT images. Therefore:

- The lymph nodes adjacent to the aorta and inferior vena cava, from vertebra T12 to the aortic bifurcation are called para-aortic.
- The lymph nodes adjacent to the common iliac vessels (from the bifurcation of the aorta to the appearance of the internal iliac arteries) are called common iliac nodes.
- The lymph nodes adjacent to the external iliac vessels and which extend anteriorly over the psoas muscle and posteriorly, including the group of obturator lymph nodes, are called external iliac lymph nodes.
- The lymph nodes adjacent to the femoral vessels at the level of the inner edge of the ischial tuberosities, are called inguinal lymph nodes.

The authors did not include internal iliac lymph nodes in their study since these are not constantly visualized by lymphangiography. They concluded with guidelines for CTV contouring:

- Addition of a 2-cm margin around the aorta, a 1-cm margin around the inferior vena cava, a 1.5-cm margin around the common iliac artery, a 2-cm margin around the external iliac artery, and a 2-cm margin around the femoral artery.
- Addition of a 1.5-cm margin medial to the iliopsoas muscle starting from intervertebral space S2–S3 and continuing until the vascular expansion volume is visualized, to include the lateral external iliac lymph nodes.
- Addition of a 1.7-cm margin medial to the pelvic wall, starting 1 cm above intervertebral space S2–S3 and continuing inferior to the inguinal nodes, to include the obturator nodes (or medial external iliac nodes).
- Exclusion of bones and air.
- Reaching to 0.5 cm from intestinal or bladder volume and 0.5 cm ventrally with respect to the aorta and the common iliac arteries.

After these studies, Portaluri et al. [91, 92] described on CT images the anatomical boundaries for each pelvic nodal chain, on the basis of CT images showing enlarged pelvic lymph nodes in cancer patients.

Moreover, as regards lymph nodes in prostatic, gynecological, bladder, and rectal cancer, Gregoire's book [6] provided explanatory contouring on CT images and a description of the related anatomical boundaries.

Table 3.4 describes the cranial, caudal, medial, lateral, anterior, and posterior anatomicoradiological boundaries of pelvic lymph nodes based on our experience.

Table 3.4 – Anatomicoradiological boundaries of pelvic region lymph nodes

Lymph nodes	Anatomical boundaries					
	Cranial	Caudal	Medial	Lateral	Anterior	Posterior
Common iliac nodes	Bifurcation of abdominal aorta (at the inferior border of L4)	Bifurcation of the common iliac vessels (at the inferior border of L5, at the level of the superior border of the ala of sacrum)	Loose cellular tissue	Psoas muscle	Loose cellular tissue anterior to the common iliac vessels	Body of L5
Internal iliac nodes	Bifurcation of common iliac vessels (at the inferior border of L5)	Plane through superior border of the head of femurs at the level of the superior border of the coccyx	Loose cellular tissue	Piriformis muscle	Posterior border of the external iliac lymph nodes and loose cellular tissue	Loose cellular tissue
External iliac nodes	Bifurcation of common iliac vessels (at the inferior border of L5)	Femoral artery	Loose cellular tissue	Iliopsoas muscle	Loose cellular tissue	Anterior border of the internal iliac lymph nodes and loose cellular tissue
Obturator nodes	Plane through the acetabulum	Superior border of the neck of femurs, at the small ischiadic foramen	Loose cellular tissue	Internal obturator muscle (intrapelvic portion)	Loose cellular tissue	Loose cellular tissue
Presacral nodes	Intervertebral space of L5–S1 (sacral promontory)	Superior border of the 1st coccygeal vertebra	–	Piriformis muscle	Loose cellular tissue	Anterior aspect of sacrum
Inguinal nodes	Superior limit of the neck of femurs	Bifurcation of the femoral artery into its superficial and deep branches	Adductor muscles	For superficial inguinal nodes: the adipose and loose connective tissue and the sartorius muscle; for deep inguinal nodes: the femoral vessels	Subcutaneous adipose tissue	Pectineal muscle

Planing CT: Technical Notes[*]

In the treatment planning of radiation therapy, the positioning and immobilization of the patient established when preparing CT simulation are especially important. For all treatment modalities, a key requirement is to place the patient in a comfortable, reproducible position that enables both irradiation of the target volume with the maximum dose and the greatest sparing of healthy tissue.

In radiation treatment planning of head and neck tumors, the patient is placed in the supine position. As a rule, a head support is provided to achieve a neutral position or, if necessary, the neck is hyperextended. Immobilization of the patient's head, neck, and shoulders in this position is usually achieved by means of a thermoplastic mask fixed to a base plate secured to the treatment table. Moreover, depending on the type of therapy to be performed, beside these, other immobilization systems can be used, such as the intraoral stent. The arms usually lie along the body, but patients may also be asked to cross their arms over their chest so as to lower their shoulders and reduce the occurrence of "beam hardening artifacts" on CT images.

In mediastinal irradiation, patients lie supine with both arms extended above the head. It is advisable to use personalized positioning and immobilization systems and controlled breathing procedures so as to minimize the geometrical uncertainty of the treatment (vacuum system, T-bar device, Perspex cast).

For treatments extended to the upper abdomen, the patient usually lies in the supine position, and an immobilization system is recommended (e.g., cast or vacuum system). Moreover, for better setup of treatment fields, the arms should be raised above the head.

In some cases of radiation delivery to the pelvic region, the prone position may be considered as an alternative to the supine position. For instance, the supine position is recommended for the treatment of anal cancer and gynecological tumors. On the other hand, rectal cancer requires a prone setup, possibly with the support of systems for displacing the small bowel (especially in the event of preoperative treatment). Radiotherapy of prostate cancer is mostly performed in the supine position, but the prone position has been reported for this tumor as well. Moreover, supports may be placed under the patient's knees to improve relaxation of the back, hindered by the rigid treatment couch. Since foot displacements can also change the relative position of bony landmarks that are crucial for determining

---

[*] This chapter has been written with the contributions of Raffaella Basilico, Antonella Filippone, Maria Luigia Storto, and Armando Tartaro

the accuracy of setup, specific "foot-blocking" supports can also be used.

As for the choice of the prone setup, it should be considered that it favors spontaneous gravitational displacement of the small bowel outside the pelvis. Another condition favoring the prone position is the difficult repositioning of treatment fields on obese patients. The skin marks on the anterior pelvic region of these patients can shift, even by several centimeters, due to the presence of adipose tissue. On the other hand, the posterior skin surface is usually more flat and less mobile, and is therefore more suitable for placing skin marks for treatment. Some obese patients have skin folds in the lower abdomen, which can cause undesirable skin reactions. These skin folds can be carefully reduced if the patient pulls up the pendulous abdomen while acquiring the prone position.

We carried out an interdisciplinary methodology developed in collaboration with radiologists to defined some practical suggestions for the execution of the CT scan for radiation treatment planning (planning CT). The CT scanning technique should be spiral and single-slice, since it affords higher resolution and provides a greater amount of volumetric information for delineation of radiotherapy target volumes compared with sequential acquisition [80, 93, 94]. It is usually performed during free breathing.

In the presence of peripheral lung tumors an optimized version of the above-mentioned procedure may be considered, by acquiring three slow CT scans (4 s per scan) obtained during quiet respiration [95].

Computed tomography includes recording of two scout views: an anteroposterior view and a laterolateral view.

Acquisition volumes for the four main anatomical regions taken into consideration in our experience can be described as follows:

- **Head-neck.** The acquisition volume can be considered to extend from a plane tangential to the upper edge of the dorsum sellae (upper limit) to a plane 2 cm caudal to the upper edge of the sternal manubrium (lower limit).
- **Mediastinum.** The acquisition volume extends from the cricoid cartilage (upper limit) to the L2 vertebra (lower limit) [80].
- **Upper abdominal region.** The acquisition volume extends from a plane located 2 cm above the liver dome (upper limit) to the level of the iliac crests (lower limit).
- **Pelvis.** The upper limit has been established 1 cm cranial to the upper limit of the iliac crests, while the lower limit is located at the level of the ischiorectal fossae or, in case of rectal cancer infiltrating the anal canal, or cancer of the anal canal, or of the vulva and vaginal canal, at the level of the anal verge.

The main parameters for the execution of CT scans in the different anatomical regions are listed in Table 4.1.

The recommended window settings for best viewing of different tissues of the four anatomical regions are the following:

- **Head-neck.** The window width and window level of CT images for head-neck soft tissues are 350 Hounsfield units (HU) and 35 HU, respectively. The corresponding settings for bone structure analysis are 2,000 HU and 400 HU.
- **Chest.** The appropriate viewing window for the mediastinum has a width of 400 HU and a level of + 40 HU, while for the pulmonary parenchyma the recommended width is 1,600 HU and level is −600 HU [96, 97].
- **Upper abdominal region.** For studying the upper abdominal region, the recommended window level is 40 HU while window width is 350–400 HU.
- **Pelvis.** For soft tissues a width of 400 HU and a level of 40 HU are recommended. For bones, recommended values are the same as for the head and neck region.

Planning CT: Technical Notes

Table 4.1 – Parameters for performing the planning CT

Head-neck	
Slice thickness	3 mm
Table speed/rotation	3 mm/s
Pitch	1
Reconstruction interval	3 mm
kV	120–130
mA	220–240
Algorithm	Soft/standard (kernel 4–6)
Matrix	512 × 512 pixel
FOV (field of view)	Adapted to the patient and sized to include the patient's contour
Mediastinum[a]	
Slice thickness	5 mm
Table speed/rotation	5–8 mm/s
Pitch	1.0–1.6
Reconstruction interval	5 mm
kV	120
mA	240
Algorithm	Soft/standard
Matrix	1,024 × 1,024 pixel
FOV	Adapted to the patient and sized to include the patient's contour
Upper abdominal region	
Slice thickness	5 mm
Table speed/rotation	8 mm/s
Pitch	1.6
Reconstruction interval	5 mm
kV	140
mA	240
Algorithm	Soft/standard
Matrix	1,024 × 1,024 pixel
FOV	Adapted to the patient and sized to include the patient's contour
Pelvis[b]	
Slice thickness	8 mm
Table speed/rotation	10 mm/s
Pitch	1.25
Reconstruction interval	5 mm
kV	140
mA	240

[a] For possible optimization of the CT acquisition method, the parameters for this region may be changed as follows: slice thickness 3 mm, table speed/rotation 3 mm/s, reconstruction interval 3 mm

[b] For possible optimization of the CT acquisition method, the parameters for this region may be changed as follows: slice thickness 5 mm, table speed/rotation 8 mm/s, reconstruction interval 4 mm

Table 4.1 – (*continued*) **Parameters for performing the planning CT**

Pelvis[b]	
Algorithm	Soft/standard
Matrix	1,024 × 1,024 pixel
FOV	Adapted to the patient and sized to include the patient's contour

[a] For possible optimization of the CT acquisition method, the parameters for this region may be changed as follows: slice thickness 3 mm, table speed/rotation 3 mm/s, reconstruction interval 3 mm

[b] For possible optimization of the CT acquisition method, the parameters for this region may be changed as follows: slice thickness 5 mm, table speed/rotation 8 mm/s, reconstruction interval 4 mm

Section II

Target Volume Delineation in Modern Radiation Therapy

5

Critical Importance of Target Definition, Including Lymph Nodes, in Image-Guided Radiation Therapy*

Exciting advances have taken place in oncology, including enhanced knowledge of molecular biology and genetics, functional imaging (positron emission tomography scanning), image-guided radiation therapy and robotic surgery, increased use of monoclonal antibodies, as well as molecular targeted cytotoxic agents, which are increasingly applied to clinical situations. At the same time there have been remarkable technological developments in radiation oncology, including the use of more powerful and versatile computers for treatment planning, radiation dose delivery, data processing, and informatics and electronic innovations coupled with sophisticated design of linear accelerators (i.e., multileaf collimators). This has resulted in an increasing use of volumetric image-based treatment planning for the delivery of radiation therapy using three-dimensional conformal radiation therapy (3DCRT), intensity modulated radiation therapy (IMRT) or image-guided radiation therapy (IGRT), stereotactic radiosurgery/radiation therapy (SRS/SRT), stereotactic body radiation therapy (SBRT), image-guided brachytherapy, radiolabeled compounds, and special particle therapy (protons, heavy ions). Computer-controlled treatment delivery systems having advanced on-board imaging, such as kilovoltage cone beam CT (kV CBCT), megavoltage (MV) helical CT, and MV electronic portal imaging, are increasingly used to enhance treatment delivery verification [98, 99].

Ling and colleagues [100] summarized imaging advances that have potential application in radiation oncology and emphasized the need to adequately identify gross, clinical, and planning target volumes as defined by International Commission on Radiation Units and Measurements (ICRU) reports 50 and 62 (Fig. 5.1). They proposed the concept of a biological target volume (BTV), which can be derived from biological images that will substantially refine target volume delineation, treatment planning, and radiation therapy delivery. They noted that, in the future, radiation therapy clinical dosimetry will incorporate both physical and biological conformity and evidence-based multidimensional conformal therapy to improve the treatment of patients with cancer using 3DCRT, IMRT, IGRT, or other techniques. Central to all these advances is the need to carefully and continuously account for anatomical variations, different tumor locations and configurations, concerns with organs at risk in the irradiated volumes, and motion of the patient or the internal target volume/organs during a course of fraction-

---

* This chapter has been written with the contributions of James A. Purdy

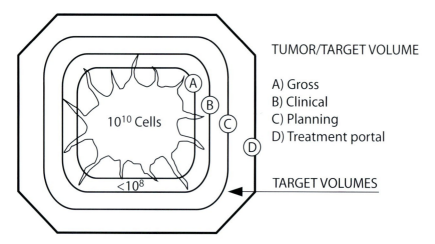

FIG. 5.1 Schematic representation of target volumes in radiation therapy treatment planning. (Reproduced with permission, Perez CA, Brady LW, Roti Roti JL (1998) Overview. In: Perez CA, Brady LW (eds) Principles and Practice of Radiation Oncology, 3rd edn. Lippincott-Raven, Philadelphia, pp 1–78)

ated radiation therapy. Strategies to address such spatial uncertainties have included elaborate patient immobilization techniques, careful simulation, accurate tumor delineation, use of margins around the tumor/clinical target volume(s), re-simulation and re-planning, and portal imaging, and more recently on-board volumetric CT imaging.

Innovations in medical imaging, including computed tomography (CT) and magnetic resonance imaging (MRI), have been invaluable in these efforts, providing a fully three-dimensional model of the patient's anatomy and the tumor volume, which is sometimes complemented with functional imaging, such as positron emission tomography (PET) or magnetic resonance spectroscopy (MRS). This advanced imaging technology allows the radiation oncologist to more accurately identify target volumes and their spatial relationship to adjacent critical normal organs. Besides the outline of the primary tumor and adjacent structures that may harbor microscopic extensions of tumor, it is critical to identify any enlarged metastatic lymph nodes and to recognize lymphatic draining regions that may be at risk for metastatic involvement (which are electively treated with a lymph node dissection or with irradiation).

The exact definition of tumor and target volumes is critical to the implementation of various approaches to image-based radiation therapy, including 3DCRT, IMRT, IGRT, and stereotactic techniques. The standard procedure for delineation of tumor volumes and organs at risk is the use of a planning CT, in most instances with contrast agents for more accurate imaging of tumors or blood vessels. However, in specific instances MRI provides better imaging of soft tissues masses. For instance, several authors have noted that delineation of the prostate can be more accurately achieved with MRI, particularly in identification of the prostatic apex [101]. Further, of equal importance is the understanding that in evaluating the prostate, as a recent study demonstrated, even radiologists trained in general MRI interpretation are not as accurate in defining the prostate as MRI experts who concentrate specifically on genitourinary MRI [102].

In defining the target volume, the radiation oncologist must appreciate the uncertainties in the target volume definition, which is dependent on the imaging modality used, the ability to fuse image sets, the capability to accurately account for the microscopic extensions, ability to account for patient immobilization uncertainties, internal target motion, and, most importantly, the individual physician's ability in assimilating all of this information, including the imaging interpretation, to perform the necessary contouring to define the target volume(s) [99].

Respiration has been shown to introduce substantial uncertainty in target positioning when irradiating patients with intrathoracic or upper abdomen tumors. Faster multislice CT scanners permit obtaining images that incorporate changes in target position which can be incorporated into the planning of radiation therapy, a process that has been called four-dimensional (4D) treatment planning [103]. Several approaches to 4D target delineation have been described [104–108] enabling reconstruction of an "internal target volume" (ITV), consisting of imaging data acquired in separate phases of respiration into a combined 3D volume containing the probable location of tumor. Allen et al. [109] created a composite volume based on the tumor delineated on maximal inhalation and exhalation scans in 16 patients. This structure was significantly smaller than a 1-cm uniform expansion around the gross tumor volume delineated on a free-breathing scan, indicating that a standard approach using a 1-cm expansion leads to overtreatment of normal tissues.

Advances in computer and electronic technology have had a major impact on the treatment planning and delivery process of radiation treatment. Medical linear accelerators and related devices come equipped with sophisticated computer-controlled multileaf collimator systems (MLCs) and integrated imaging systems that provide beam aperture and/or beam-intensity modulation capabilities which allow precise shaping and positioning of actually delivered radiation dose distributions in the patient [110].

It should be clearly understood that modern-day radiation oncology treatment outcomes are very much dependent on the computer models and algorithms used, as they impact definition of target volumes, organs at risk, optimal dose distributions, dose-volume statistics, the determination of tumor control possibility (TCP), the normal tissue complication probability (NTCP), and other biological parameters related to treatment planning and delivery [99].

5.1 Target Volume and Critical Structure Delineation

The definition of target volumes and organs at risk has been standardized following the nomenclature published in the ICRU reports 50 and 62. Macroscopic or known tumor is designated as gross tumor volume (GTV), suspected microscopic spread as clinical target volume (CTV), and marginal volumes necessary to account for both setup variations and organ and patient motion are designated as planning target volume (PTV) (Fig. 5.1) [98].

While the current recommendations direct the radiation oncologist to specifically account for microscopic disease uncertainty, and patient setup and organ movement uncertainties in defining the PTVs, it must be recognized that with current technology this is in reality still a judgment call and not an exact science for most cases. In performing this task, the radiation oncologist must rely on his/her experience and judgment drawn from study of the literature, and observation and evaluation of patients treated regarding risk of failure versus normal tissue complications. In other words, when confronted with the problem of defining the volume to receive a prescribed dose, or defining an organ at risk in order to avoid or limit the dose, the radiation oncologist must make a series of trade-offs.

The reproducibility and accuracy of GTV delineation for most treatment sites is generally not very well known, as it is based mostly on clinical judgment. It is known that the shape and size of the GTV can depend significantly on the imaging modality

[101, 111]. Leunens et al. [112] reported that they observed a considerable intra- and interobserver variation in GTV delineation for brain tumors. Ten Haken et al. [113] and Rasch et al. [114] compared GTVs defined using both CT and MRI; in both reports, the target volume defined using CT and MRI was different than the volume defined using CT alone. Furthermore, Rasch et al. [115] concluded that MRI-derived target volumes had less interobserver variation than CT only derived target volumes. In another study, Roach et al. [101] compared the delineated prostate volumes using both CT and MRI for a series of patients and found significant volume differences in approximately one third of the cases, depending on the imaging modality used.

In 2008, CT is still the principal source of imaging data used for defining the GTV for 3DCRT and IMRT treatment planning for most sites, but this imaging modality presents several potential pitfalls. First, when contouring the GTV, it is essential that the appropriate CT window and level settings be used in order to determine the maximum dimension of what is considered potential gross disease. Secondly, for those treatment sites in which there is considerable organ motion, such as for tumors in the thorax, CT images do not correctly represent either the time-averaged position of the tumor or its true shape. This is due to the fact that the current CT simulation process relies almost exclusively on the use of fast, spiral CT technology, and thus acquires data essentially in two dimensions (2D). This has the effect of capturing the tumor cross-section images at particular positions in the breathing cycle. Caldwell et al. [116] studied this problem showing that if the tumor motion is large, different, and possibly non-contiguous, transverse sections of the tumor could be imaged at different points of the breathing cycle, leading to volume uncertainties. They pointed out that the interpolation process in spiral CT technology adds further to the uncertainty and concluded that 3D reconstruction of the GTV from temporally variant 2D images will contain distortions that are not only non-representative of the true geometry of the stationary tumor but also are not a good representation of the tumor and its motion. In their study, they further concluded that PET imaging could provide a more accurate representation of the GTV encompassing motion of such tumors and thus has the potential to provide patient-specific motion volumes for an individualized ITV. There is no quick solution to this problem. Perhaps when multislice CT technology (so-called 4D CT imaging) becomes the standard for CT simulation the problem will be minimized. Until then, however, one must be very careful when defining a GTV using CT images only in those cases where the tumor motion is significant.

Unfortunately, in many sites anatomical imaging techniques (i.e., CT or MRI) do not always distinguish malignant from normal tissues. Thus, there is growing interest in incorporating the complementary information available from functional imaging, such as PET, when defining the GTV [100, 117, 118].

Functional images show metabolic, physiological, genotypic, and phenotypic data that may improve the staging of patients with cancer and target definition for radiation therapy. Major accomplishments have taken place in functional imaging with various radionuclides, and development is underway on methods that will characterize the genotype and phenotype of tumors by non-invasive molecular imaging technology.

Positron emission tomography scanning measures in vivo biochemical disturbances (such as accelerated glucose metabolism) associated with malignant neoplasms. Deoxy-glucose labeled with fluorine (F18-FDG) is frequently used to assess functional tumor biology and metabolism. After FDG is intravenously injected, its uptake in tissues is measured for approximately 60 min with PET scanning. FDG is transported to the membrane of the cell; increasing the number of glucose transport molecules at the surface of the tumor cell will enhance glucose and FDG uptake. Intercellular hexokinase will convert FDG into FDG-6-phosphate, which exists at low levels in tumor cells. Because the deoxy component of FDG blocks further degradation of FDG-6-phosphate, FDG phosphate accumulates in the cell and emits positrons. The distribution of the FDG reflects the level of glucose consumption at a specific site. The minimal size of lesions detected on PET scan is 3–5 mm depending on the location of the lesion, uptake of the radionuclide, and the activity of the surrounding tissues. Clinical applications of PET scanning in oncology include: (1) differentiating benign from malignant lesions (albeit, not always accurately), (2) staging of malignant tumors, (3) treatment planning including radiation therapy, and (4) monitoring treatment results and follow-up [119, 120].

Gregoire [121], in an editorial, pointed out the increasing use of PET scanning to determine tumor extent and as a guide for radiation therapy treatment planning in patients with cancer, spearheaded by the popularity of 3DCRT and IMRT. He thoughtfully discussed issues related to sensitivity and specificity of PET scanning in different anatomical locations, which affect the usefulness of this modality in clinical practice. The advent of integrated PET/CT devices markedly facilitates the acquisition of anatomically and physiologically fused images under similar conditions for radiation therapy treatment planning. This comprehensive review is highly recommended for those interested in this technology. In the future it will be possible to expand the applications of PET in oncology by taking advantage of in vivo distribution of radionuclides such as ^{15}O, ^{11}C, and others mentioned in this review. Similarly, single photon emission tomography (SPECT) can be used to quantify in vivo distribution of receptor targeting compounds labeled with ^{111}In, ^{99m}Tc, or ^{123}I.

Bourguet and Groupe de Travail Standards, Options and Recommendations Project [122] reviewed 600 articles identified in Medline, web sites, and personal reference lists of expert members and submitted them for review to independent reviewers and developed guidelines for the use of FDG-PET scanning in the diagnosis of the primary tumor, treatment response, and examination for recurrence. The recommendations were made on the basis of data published up to February 2002. Systematic monitoring of the new scientific data on FDG-PET was set up to ensure updating of available reports.

The ultimate goal of radiation therapy treatment planning is to biologically characterize and accurately delineate the target volume, plan an effective course of therapy, predict tumor and normal tissue response (TCP, NTCP), and monitor the outcome of treatment. Functional imaging may significantly contribute to achieving these objectives. For example, Caldwell et al. reported high observer variability in CT-based definition of the GTV for non-small cell lung cancer patients when compared with the GTV defined using FDG-hybrid PET images co-registered with CT [123]. Another example of the use of functional imaging in target volume definition is provided by Chao et al. in which they proposed the use of PET employing a hypoxic tumor-specific tracer to define the hypoxic region of the GTV for potentially guiding IMRT treatment delivery [124].

If PET or other modality imaging studies are used to complement the CT planning process, they must be accurately registered to the planning CT data set [125–127]. While significant improvements in radiation therapy planning (RTP) fusion software have been made, image registration remains one of the serious pitfalls that can befall the radiation oncologist when defining the GTV [128, 129]. The radiation oncologist and treatment planner must be especially vigilant when using multiple imaging studies when defining volumes and be sure that robust quality assurance (QA) processes are in place.

Delineating the CTV is a more complicated task than delineating either the GTV or most organs at risk. At this time, it is more of an art than a science since current imaging techniques are not capable of detecting subclinical tumor involvement directly. When defining GTV/CTVs and organs at risk on axial CT slices, assistance from a diagnostic radiologist is often helpful. Publications addressing the problem of establishing a consistent CTV for various clinical sites are now becoming more common [26, 72]. Research efforts that will allow a more accurate determination of CTV is an important area to further advance radiation therapy treatment planning.

Specifying the margins around the CTV to create the PTV is also not an exact science. The treating physician should take into account data from published literature and/or any uncertainty studies performed in their clinic. A recent review by Langen and Jones [105] provides the most comprehensive compilation of organ motion data to date. Interfraction organ motion studies have focused mainly on the treatment of prostate cancer [130–133]. Intrafraction motion studies have focused on variations caused by respiratory motion for disease in the thoracic and upper abdominal regions [134, 135]. How to use target organ mobility and setup error data to determine the appropriate margin between the CTV and PTV is discussed later. However, it should be understood that the margin used to create the PTV should not just be based strictly on geometric uncertainty considerations. The physician must also take into account the presence of nearby organs at risk, and thus the margins used are the result of trade-offs that balance concerns for potential geometric miss versus the possibility of unacceptable toxicity.

The asymmetrical nature of the GTV/CTV geometric uncertainties must also be addressed when defining the PTV. For example, organ motion for the prostate gland has been shown to be anisotropic. Daily setup errors may also be anisotropic as side-to-side or rotational shifts of patients are likely to be different from setup differences in the anteroposterior direction.

Another concern is the fact that some 3DRTP systems still do not possess accurate methods for providing a true 3D margin around the GTV/CTV when delineating the PTV. For large contour differences in the GTV/CTV in neighboring slices, a margin expansion drawn or specified in 2D around the GTV/CTV contour will result in margins that are too small in the cranial-caudal direction. Bedford and Shentall [136] described methods to compute 3D target volume margins resolving this problem. One must understand the method used on the RTP system, and if it is based on a 2D algorithm, one should use a larger contour in the adjoining slice and cap the GTV/CTV inferiorly and superiorly.

Another potential pitfall occurs in those cases where the PTV extends outside the patient's skin contour (e.g., PTV for tangential irradiation of the breast, or for some head and neck cancer sites). In such cases, part of the PTV will have an air-like density causing an artifact in the dose distribution calculated and displayed. For practical purposes, one must change the density used for that part of the PTV in the RTP system to unity, or require the PTV margin to coincide with the skin surface. Neither method is totally correct, but regardless it is important that the treating physician be aware of the approximation used when setting or approving field margins and evaluating the dose distribution.

A serious limitation currently present with some IMRT planning systems occurs when a PTV overlaps with an organ at risk or its associated PRV. For such systems, the overlapping voxels can be assigned to only one of the volumes, typically the target volume, thus truncating the overlapping organ at risk volume (e.g., a PTV that overlaps a parotid gland). In such cases, dose-volume histogram (DVH) evaluation for the organ at risk is compromised, as is the digital data export of the contour data to centralized quality assurance centers. Concentric PTVs ($PTV_{HighDose}$ and $PTV_{LowDose}$) present this same type of limitation for these RTP systems. Thus, it is essential that the physician and the physicist fully understand the IMRT planning system's method (and limitations) used in assigning voxels, both for DVH evaluation and digital data export.

We now return to the problem of creating the margin between the CTV and PTV using organ motion and setup error data. The ICRU report 62 states that a quadratic approach similar to that recommended by the *Bureau International des Poids et Mesures* (BIPM) can be used. Antolak and Rosen concluded that to insure that every point on the edge of the CTV be within the PTV approximately 95% of the time, the CTV should be expanded using a normalized radius of expansion of 1.65 times the SD in each direction [137]. Van Herk et al. [138] calculated probability distributions of the cumulative dose over a population of patients (which they called dose-population histograms) and studied the effects of random and systematic geometric deviations on the cumulative dose distribution to the CTV. Margin recipes to create the PTV could be obtained from a single point on this type of histogram. Craig et al. [139] concluded that a coverage of about 95% is a reasonable goal for PTV design and that geometric uncertainties from different sources should be added in quadrature, unless there are compelling reasons to do otherwise.

To better clarify the sources of geometric uncertainties, the Netherlands Cancer Institute group [138] has suggested dividing them into uncertainties that occur during treatment preparation (systematic errors) and those that occur daily during treatment execution (random variations). Treatment execution uncertainties include the interfraction variations (i.e., day to day variation in the patient setup or equipment), and also the intrafraction variations (i.e., movement of the patient or GTV/CTV within a single fraction). Treatment preparation uncertainties include setup error and organ motion on the planning CT simulator study, delineation errors, and equipment calibration errors. They suggest that the effects of execution errors can be estimated during treatment planning by blurring (i.e., convolving) the computed dose distribution with the known error distribution and ensuring that the blurred dose distribution conforms to the PTV [138]. Van Herk et al. [140] pointed out that a limitation of many previous studies addressing this area is the fact that either only execution uncertainties were evaluated, or at most only a few of the preparation uncertainties were included. They pointed out that because preparation errors have a much larger impact on the target dose than execution errors, the effect of excluding preparation errors in tumor control probability (TCP) evaluation is that very small margins can appear to be adequate. They conclude that preparation errors may in fact play the most important role, as such small margins will lead to frequent geometric misses.

Yu et al. [141] were one of the first to report on the effects of intrafraction organ motion on the delivery of IMRT noting that unlike static field treatments, where intrafraction organ motion only affects the boundaries creating a broader dose penumbra, the interplay of the movement of the MLC produced beamlets and the movement of the patient anatomy can create "hot" and "cold" spots throughout the field. They concluded that interfraction effects could cause the magnitude of intensity variations in the target to be greater than ±50% from the calculated values without motion, but noted that intensity variations were strongly dependent on the speed of the beam aperture relative to the speed of the target motion, and the width of the scanning beam relative to the amplitude of target motion. They suggested that the speed of collimator motion be kept as slow as possible, and that the gap between the two opposing MLC leaves be kept as large as possible. They pointed out that for a given desired intensity distribution, the above two requirements may be in conflict and some form of optimization may be required.

Such studies have reinforced the concern about using IMRT for the treatment of moving CTVs and raised the question whether the PTV concept is applicable to IMRT. Such concerns have helped spur the development of tumor tracking and respiratory gating technologies [142, 143]. Bortfeld et al. [144] has also addressed this issue of intrafraction organ motion and the delivery of IMRT and pointed out that because IMRT treatments are typically delivered over about 30 treatment fractions, and not in a single session, there will be some averaging over the course of treatment, and the relative cumulative error after several fractions will most likely be much smaller than the error on a single day. They concluded that any additional effects that are specific to the IMRT delivery technique appear to be relatively small, except for a scanning beam type IMRT. More studies addressing the issue of intrafraction organ motion during the delivery of IMRT are still warranted.

All of the issues discussed point out that the PTV/PRV concept simplifies accounting for geometric uncertainties but does give rise to several dilemmas. Particularly important is the loss of actual tumor and normal organ volumes information for researchers developing TCP and normal tissue complication (NTCP) models. While it does not appear possible to totally eliminate the PTV concept at this time, it does appear possible to use smaller margins for some sites if more frequent imaging or other technical innovation is used to reduce geometric uncertainties. For example, for prostate cancer, the use of daily ultrasound imaging, or daily electronic portal imaging of implanted radiopaque markers, to relocate the target volume with reference to the machine's isocenter does allow for a smaller margin for the PTV [130, 145]. However, one must still be prudent in the amount of margin reduction when using these technologies.

For treatment sites in the thorax, ways to minimize respiratory motion and its effects include the use of ventilation-based gating, breath-holding, and active breathing control [142, 146–148]. The different methods include various tradeoffs ranging from treatment machine control, which is not dependent on the patient, to systems that are completely dependent on the patient. Again, regardless of which technique is used to reduce the overall PTV margin, one must be prudent in the amount of margin reduction.

Yan et al. [149–151] proposed an individual patient-based approach for determining PTV (called adaptive radiation therapy), as opposed to the current situation of using population-based averages of the setup errors or organ motion. In this approach, early measurements (multiple CT scans and daily portal images) during the first few patient treatments are performed to determine the required margins for later treatments based on the localization data for the individual patient. An extension of this approach is the current use of daily (or weekly) CT images obtained on the treatment machine to ascertain the anatomy of the patient and the location and deformable contours of the target and organs at risk to provide feedback that is used to modify the treatment plan and delivery of the irradiation, resulting on a more precise dose distribution.

Yan and Lockman [151] have pointed out that the temporal dose-volume variation brought on by fractionated radiation therapy is not presently accounted for in any reporting schemes, i.e., the location of the organ/tumor/patient during a course of radiation therapy varies with respect to the radiation beams. In other words, the temporal variation of each tissue voxel irradiated is currently not taken into account, causing uncertainties in understanding the tumor and normal tissue dose response, thereby limiting reliable treatment evaluation and optimization. Improved models that account for organ deformation and movements will be needed to address this important issue.

One final practical issue should be clearly understood by the treatment planner. Once the PTV has been defined, additional margin beyond the PTV is needed when designing the beam portal in order to obtain dose coverage because of beam penumbra related to treatment technique. Typically, a 7- to 9-mm margin (port edge to PTV) is generally a good starting point for 3DCRT techniques, but one should consider the actual characteristics of the beams used to make this starting point determination. Also, in the case of coplanar treatment techniques, the margins required across the axial plane of treatment and the margins orthogonal to this plane will be different. For example, a larger inferior-superior portal margin is always needed for coplanar techniques to ensure that the prescribed isodose surface covers the PTV. Also, in many situations, the lateral and anterior-posterior portal margins for each field can be reduced (providing better organ at risk sparing) by adjusting each beam's relative weighting. It should be clear that making a hard rule about margin sizes is unrealistic and requires some planning iteration to find the best mix of superior-inferior, anterior-posterior, lateral margins, and beam weights. The ability of IMRT to reduce beam margin by increasing fluence at the PTV periphery is a significant advantage of this technique in achieving PTV dose coverage while improving the sparing of adjacent organs at risk [152].

5.2 Delineation of Lymph Node Volumes

The definition of lymph node target volumes is critical in radiation therapy treatment planning, as many of these structures may or are involved by a variety of malignant tumors in many anatomical locations.

In patients with head and neck cancer, careful studies using CT scans have identified the location of metastatic lymph nodes, including the retropharyngeal nodes in carcinoma of the oropharynx, which were present in 16% of 208 patients and in 23% of those with nodal disease in other neck sites [153]. Further, a more precise location of the lymph nodes will aid in better defining the margins required to adequately cover the nodal target volumes in patients with carcinoma of the oropharynx, hypopharynx, or larynx (Fig. 5.2) [154, 155]. Gregoire et al. [26], Nowak et al. [67], and Chao et al. [74], the latter based on a study correlating patterns of failure in 126 patients with head and neck cancer, developed guidelines for nodal target volume delineation.

In the thorax, Yuan et al. [156] evaluated extracapsular tumor extension in 243 patients with non-small cell lung cancer (noted in 41% of the patients and 33.4% of the lymph nodes) and made recommendations for CTV margins as a function of the size of the lymph nodes. Chapet et al. [83] generated a 3D radiological description for hilar and mediastinal nodes, based on axial CT scans of the thorax, which, as in this book, will be of great value in defining target volumes in radiation treatment planning. Steenbakkers et al. [157] illustrated the geometric uncertainties that exist when CT scans are used for lung cancer target delineation and how this can be improved using PET scanning. Other authors have documented the value of PET scanning in determining target volumes in patients with lung cancer (Fig. 5.3) [158, 159].

Brunner et al. [160] in 175 patients with pancreatic cancer who underwent pancreatoduodenectomy assessed regional and para-aortic nodal spread, using CT scans, identified regional node metastasis in 76% and in distant nodes in 22%. Based on this data standardized treatment planning recommendations were developed.

In the pelvis, lymphangiography was used to generate 3D lymph node mapping for treatment planning in 16 patients with cervical cancer [90]. Also, iliopelvic lymphoscintigraphy (with 99 m technetium nanocolloids) was shown to have sensitivity ranging from 40% for presacral and hypogastric nodes to 70–80% for external, common iliac, and para-aortic nodes to 100% for inguinal nodes in 70 patients [161] and pelvic CT scans were used to identify in 3D images lymph nodes in 20 patients with various pelvic malignancies [92]. Finlay et al. [162] contoured the pelvic arteries on CT scans of 43 patients with cervical cancer. The vessel contours were hidden, conventional pelvic irradiation fields were outlined, and coverage of lymph node regions was analyzed. Superiorly 34 patients (79%) had inadequate coverage; on the AP field in 9 (21%) and in the lateral field in 30 (70%) patients margins were also inadequate.

In 18 patients with prostate cancer who had pathologically confirmed node-positive disease, Shih et al. [108] using a novel magnetic resonance

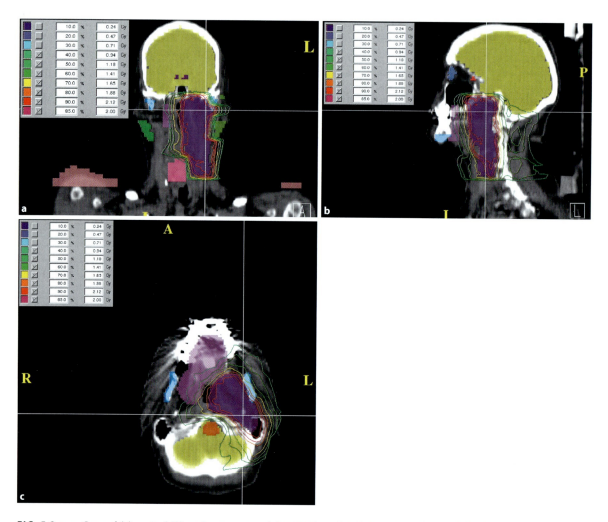

FIG. 5.2 a–c Coronal (**a**), sagittal (**b**), and cross-section (**c**) IMRT dose distributions for patient with head and neck cancer

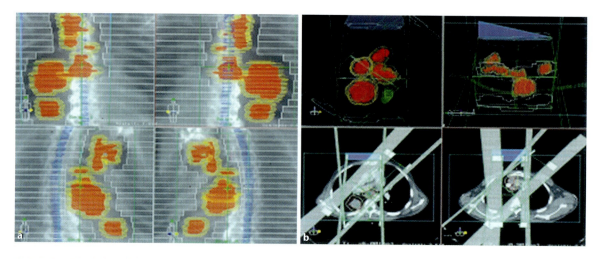

FIG. 5.3 a Simulation of thorax in a patient with carcinoma of the left lung with mediastinal lymph nodes detected on PET scan. **b** Illustration of 3DCRT plan in patient with carcinoma of the lung

lymphangiographic nanoparticle technique highlighted the likely metastatic sites. To reduce the volume of pelvic organs irradiated they proposed a pelvic CTV to encompass regions at high risk of harboring occult nodal metastasis to include a 2-cm radial expansion around the common and proximal external and internal iliac vessels that would encompass 94.5% of the pelvic nodes at risk in patients with node-positive prostate cancer.

Precise imaging of the pelvic and para-aortic lymph nodes in gynecological cancer and the advent of IMRT has facilitated the irradiation of these regional lymphatics while sparing the small intestine and pelvic organs (Fig. 5.4).

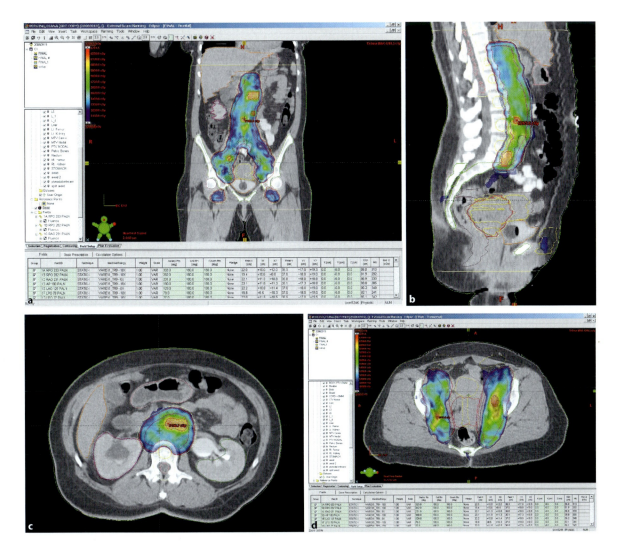

FIG. 5.4 a Representation of dose distribution with IMRT for irradiation of para-aortic and pelvic lymph nodes in patient with carcinoma of the uterine cervix. **b** Sagittal representation of same dose distributions. **c** Cross-section dose distribution of above. **d** Cross-section of IMRT dose distribution for irradiation of pelvic lymphatics in patient with carcinoma of uterine cervix

5.3 Implications of Target Definition for Innovative Technology in Contemporary Radiation Therapy

With the advent of new and more complex technology, such as cone beam [163–165], tomotherapy [166–168], robotic radiation therapy, etc., and the increasing use of image-based radiation therapy [169], including 3D conformal, IMRT, both cranial and extracranial stereotactic [170] and adaptive radiation therapy [171], in many instances using single fraction or hypofractionated irradiation schedules [172] with more tightly defined margins around the target volumes, it is critical to more accurately delineate not only the primary target but also lymphatic volumes at risk for metastatic spread. More precise and versatile algorithms for treatment planning are mandatory to enhance the opportunities for dose optimization with these technologies.

Furthermore, more precise treatment delivery techniques are required to ensure accurate delivery of the irradiation, including ultrasound, portal imaging devices, and methods for tracking the position of the target during treatment, such as the Calypso system with radiofrequency transponders implanted in the target volume, to decrease the errors that may be introduced by intrafraction motion of the target or the organs at risk [173–175].

A concern that has been expressed by some, with the use of IMRT or scatter-foil proton generators, is the somewhat larger volume of normal tissues of the patient that receives low doses of irradiation, which potentially may result in an increase in second malignancies [176]. Aoyama et al. [177] noted that the dose of irradiation to unwanted tissues is lower with tomotherapy compared to IMRT.

5.4 Quality Assurance

While this chapter has focused on the critical importance of accurate target volume definition, it must be understood that this task is one of many that quality assurance programs must address. To ensure the quality of radiation therapy it is mandatory to implement programs that test the functionality of the equipment and the precision of dose calibration, treatment planning, dose calculations, and delivery used in the treatment of the patient. Dosimetric quality assurance compares measured and calculated dose distributions for specific test treatment plans. The American Association of Physicists in Medicine (AAPM) and the European Society for Treatment and Research Organization (ESTRO) have published detailed reports describing acceptance testing, commissioning, and procedures for periodic quality assurance procedures of hardware and software used in radiation therapy facilities [178, 179]. Other elements of quality assurance include protocols and manuals documenting the operating procedures in the radiation facility, appropriate clinical and physics records, chart review sessions, and audits of parameters of treatment and dose verification, with participation of radiation oncologists, physicists, dosimetrists, therapists, and other personnel to ensure the proposed treatment is being accurately carried out.

Because in general the margins around the target volume are smaller and the dose gradient steeper it is necessary to exercise more care in the treatment of the patient with 3DCRT, IMRT, or IGRT. Therefore a quality assurance program for these modalities must be more detailed and demanding, as it involves not only all of the elements described above but also performance of the MLC leaf accuracy (for IMRT submillimeter accuracy is needed, speed, etc.) and the radiation output with the accelerator gantry in motion [180].

For IMRT treatment, a specific patient-directed quality assurance program is mandatory, including irradiation of anatomical phantoms with the proposed treatment parameters, using ionization chambers, film dosimetry (radiographic, radiochromic), thermoluminescent dosimeters, etc., and comparing these data with the dose distributions and DVHs generated by the treatment planning system. To determine the spatial accuracy of the treatment planning and delivery systems, the location in space of the measured and calculated doses must be precisely and independently verified. A characteristic of IMRT is a lack of convenient portal imaging to verify patient position and accuracy of dose distribution, for example, the patient position is checked with orthogonal films (anterior-posterior and lateral centered on the central axis of the multiple beam arrangement) and the images are compared to similar geometry on digitally reconstructed radiographs (DRRs). Treatment and dose distribution verification is carried out using phantoms and direct measurements [180–184].

There are numerous problems in assuring target position validity caused by both extrinsic and intrinsic factors. The intrinsic or inherent problems include the difficulties caused by the motion of the target volume (e.g., prostate) relative to the bony anatomy and adjacent organs (bladder, rectum) which has been reported by numerous authors. A target volume such as the prostate and seminal vesicles can move inferiorly, superiorly, anteriorly, posteriorly, and even rotate along the axis. In addition, respiratory motion adds another influence to these motions. In addition, there are (preparation) extrinsic errors, which are related to the actual simulation process, the definition of the target, etc. There are also execution errors, which include the inaccuracies in positioning of the patient for daily treatment. These all add to the possibilities of movement and inaccuracy in the defining of the target. The inherent movements of the prostate can be as much as 4–5 mm in certain directions, and may total as much as 10 mm. These uncertainties must be incorporated in the design of the PTV in the treatment plan (Fig. 5.5).

Motion of the organ and the patient leads to blurring of dose distribution; this can cause an increased beam penumbra. Such movements can lead to the tumor being displaced so that 10% of the volume may be out of the field 20% of the time so that the tumor is only in the actual treatment field 80% of the time. These inaccuracies have the potential to create hot and cold spots. Needless to say these cold spots and hot spots are not usually visualized in the planning process [185, 186].

Another problem is a dramatic drop in the probability level of reaching an acceptable minimum dose as the CTV margin is reduced. If a very tight margin is defined, i.e., zero margin or a few millimeters, the probability of delivering the planned high dose to the CTV approaches zero. This variation of dose around the CTV is such that only zero error will lead to the planned dose. The probability of zero error in this situation is extremely small, so this must be a concern when a very tight margin is used.

Of utmost importance is the determination of the most appropriate treatment modality for the various sites, i.e., selecting whether 3DCRT, IMRT, or IGRT is to be used. This selection depends on location of the tumor, homogeneity criteria required, the cost, the time, and the clinical outcome analysis. It is of importance to examine the difference in the dosimetry between 3DCRT and IMRT and to evaluate treatment morbidity when comparing 3DCRT to IMRT.

5.5 Cost Benefit and Utility

There is a substantial financial investment in the acquisition of modern radiation therapy treatment planning systems and devices, in addition to the documented increased time and effort involved in the procedures necessary to maintain, operate the equipment, and treat a patient with 3DCRT, IMRT, IGRT (including tomotherapy). As noted, there is significantly greater involvement of the radiation oncologist and physicist as well as more time required of the dosimetrist(s) and radiation therapists to supervise, generate, verify treatment planning, and delivery. The complexity of the treatment tech-

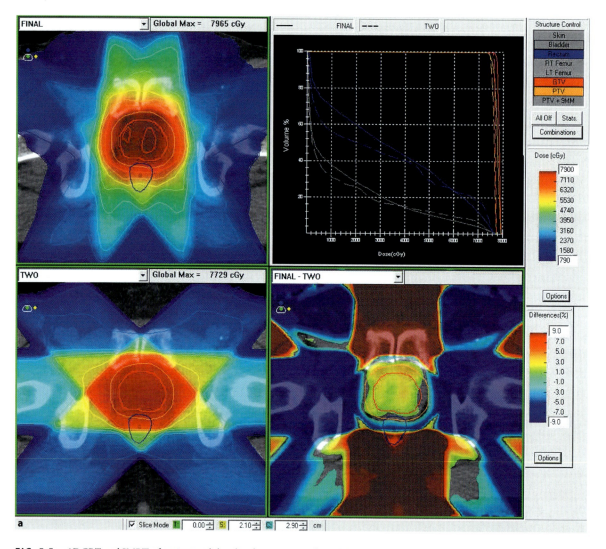

FIG. 5.5 a 3DCRT and IMRT of patient with localized carcinoma of prostate.

niques and the potential for errors that will undermine the therapeutic objectives and jeopardize the wellbeing of the patient demand more training and continuing education for all professionals involved in the management of patients treated with these modalities.

Several publications [187] have documented the time and effort of modern radiation therapy which is only partially impacted by increased experience and proficiency of the staff. In the USA this has been reflected with reimbursement for services that attempt to cover the greater use of equipment, facilities, and human resources involved in the treatment of these patients. Further, as these modalities are frequently used in conjunction with cytotoxic or molecular targeted therapies that enhance the effect of irradiation, the overall management of the patient is more complex and time consuming.

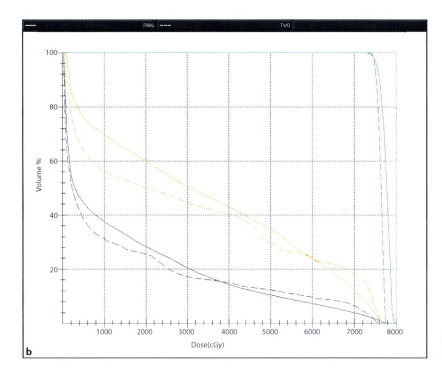

FIG. 5.5 (*continued*) **b** Dose-volume histogram of same patient

On the other hand, innovative radiation therapy and dose optimization, with more precise coverage of the target volume and delivery of higher irradiation doses with acceptable treatment morbidity has been documented to increase local-regional tumor control, survival with decreased incidence of distant metastasis, and better quality of life of the patient. Pollack et al. [188] and in an update of a randomized study comparing 70 Gy delivered with a conventional technique or 78 Gy with 3DCRT in localized carcinoma of the prostate documented improved outcome in the patients treated with the higher dose. Perez and collaborators [187] in a study of patients with localized carcinoma of the prostate noted that the re-treatment of a patient who has a tumor recurrence after initial treatment increases the total cost of therapy by about three to four times the cost of a patient treated successfully at initial treatment. Moreover, the cost of management of complications of treatment will also add to the overall cost of management of the patient.

As stated by Suit [189] "the history of medicine has repeatedly demonstrated that the perceived increased efficacy and not the cost, primarily determine the fate of new technologies."

5.6 Conclusions

Remarkable advances are evolving in radiation therapy technology that optimize the treatment of patients with cancer, with irradiation alone or combined with other modalities (surgery, chemotherapy, hormones, or biologically targeted therapies). The increased complexity of this technology requires more rigorous training of all professionals involved in the radiation therapy process and more detailed and accurate quality assurance procedures to ensure an optimal treatment of our patients.

Accurate delineation of tumor, target volumes, and organs at risk is crucial to the quality of treatment planning and delivery accomplished with innovative technologies in radiation therapy. Quality assurance in all components of the treatment planning, delivery, and verification will ensure optimal patient care and better treatment outcome.

There is an increased cost in the application of innovative techniques, but in the long run this is compensated by a lower cost in the overall treatment of a patient, as additional management of initial treatment failures or complications is threefold higher than the cost of successful and uncomplicated initial treatment.

Section III

Axial CT Radiological Anatomy

Head and Neck Lymph Nodes

* This chapter has been written with the contributions of Antonietta Augurio, Angelo Di Pilla, and Armando Tartaro

A Guide for Delineation of Lymph Nodal Clinical Target Volume in Radiation Therapy

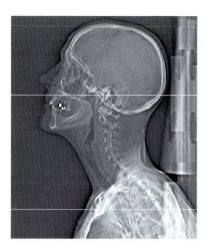

SCOUT VIEW OF HEAD AND NECK REGION

Level	Anatomical boundaries					
	Cranial	Caudal	Medial	Lateral	Anterior	Posterior
Ia	Geniohyoid m., plane tangent to basilar edge of mandible	Plane tangent to body of hyoid bone	n.a.[a]	Medial edge of ant. belly of digastric m.	Symphysis menti, platysma m.	Body of hyoid bone[b]
Ib	Mylohyoid m., cranial edge of submandibular gland	Plane through central part of hyoid bone	Lateral edge of ant. belly of digastric m.	Basilar edge/inner side of mandible, platysma m., skin	Symphysis menti, platysma m.	Posterior edge of submandibular gland
IIa	Caudal edge of lateral process of C1	Caudal edge of the body of hyoid bone	Medial edge of int. carotid artery, paraspinal (levator scapulae) m.	Medial edge of sternocleidomastoid m.	Post. edge of submandibular gland; ant. edge of int. carotid artery; post. edge of post. belly of digastric m.	Post. border of int. jugular vein
IIb	Caudal edge of lateral process of C1	Caudal edge of the body of hyoid bone	Medial edge of int. carotid artery, paraspinal (levator scapulae) m.	Medial edge of sternocleidomastoid m.	Post. border of int. jugular vein	Post. border of the sternocleidomastoid m.
III	Caudal edge of the body of hyoid bone	Caudal edge of cricoid cartilage	Int. edge of carotid artery, paraspinal (scalene) m.	Medial edge of sternocleidomastoid m.	Posterolateral edge of the sternohyoid m.; ant. edge of sternocleidomastoid m.	Post. edge of the sternocleidomastoid m.
IV	Caudal edge of cricoid cartilage	2 cm cranial to sternoclavicular joint	Medial edge of int. carotid artery, paraspinal (scalene) m.	Medial edge of sternocleidomastoid m.	Anteromedial edge of sternocleidomastoid m.	Post. edge of the sternocleidomastoid m.
V	Cranial edge of body of hyoid bone	CT slice encompassing the transverse cervical vessels[c]	Paraspinal (levator scapulae, splenius capitis) m.	Platysma m., skin	Post. edge of the sternocleidomastoid m.	Anterolateral border of the trapezius m.
VI	Caudal edge of body of thyroid cartilage[d]	Sternal manubrium	n.a.	Medial edges of thyroid gland, skin and anteromedial edge of sternocleidomastoid m.	Skin; platysma m.	Separation between trachea and esophagus[e]
RP	Base of skull	Cranial edge of the body of hyoid bone	Midline	Medial edge of int. carotid artery	Fascia under the pharyngeal mucosa	Prevertebral m. (longus colli, longus capitis)

[a] Midline structure lying between the medial borders of the anterior bellies of the digastric muscles
[b] The insertion of the thyroid muscle is often interposed between level Ia and the body of the hyoid bone
[c] For NPC, the reader is referred to the original description of the UICC/AJCC 1997 edition of the Ho's triangle. In essence, the fatty planes below and around the clavicle down to the trapezius muscle
[d] For paratracheal and recurrent nodes, the cranial border is the caudal edge of the cricoid cartilage
[e] For pretracheal nodes, trachea and anterior edge of cricoid cartilage

Source: Modified from Gregoire V, Levendag P, Ang KK, et al. (2003) [78]

A Guide for Delineation of Lymph Nodal Clinical Target Volume in Radiation Therapy

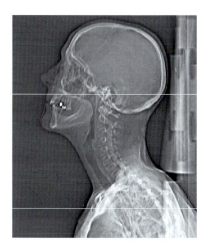

SCOUT VIEW OF HEAD AND NECK REGION

Level	Anatomical boundaries					
	Cranial	Caudal	Medial	Lateral	Anterior	Posterior
Ia	Geniohyoid m., plane tangent to basilar edge of mandible	Plane tangent to body of hyoid bone	n.a.[a]	Medial edge of ant. belly of digastric m.	Symphysis menti, platysma m.	Body of hyoid bone[b]
Ib	Mylohyoid m., cranial edge of submandibular gland	Plane through central part of hyoid bone	Lateral edge of ant. belly of digastric m.	Basilar edge/inner side of mandible, platysma m., skin	Symphysis menti, platysma m.	Posterior edge of submandibular gland
IIa	Caudal edge of lateral process of C1	Caudal edge of the body of hyoid bone	Medial edge of int. carotid artery, paraspinal (levator scapulae) m.	Medial edge of sternocleidomastoid m.	Post. edge of submandibular gland; ant. edge of int. carotid artery; post. edge of post. belly of digastric m.	Post. border of int. jugular vein
IIb	Caudal edge of lateral process of C1	Caudal edge of the body of hyoid bone	Medial edge of int. carotid artery, paraspinal (levator scapulae) m.	Medial edge of sternocleidomastoid m.	Post. border of int. jugular vein	Post. border of the sternocleidomastoid m.
III	Caudal edge of the body of hyoid bone	Caudal edge of cricoid cartilage	Int. edge of carotid artery, paraspinal (scalene) m.	Medial edge of sternocleidomastoid m.	Posterolateral edge of the sternohyoid m.; ant. edge of sternocleidomastoid m.	Post. edge of the sternocleidomastoid m.
IV	Caudal edge of cricoid cartilage	2 cm cranial to sternoclavicular joint	Medial edge of int. carotid artery, paraspinal (scalene) m.	Medial edge of sternocleidomastoid m.	Anteromedial edge of sternocleidomastoid m.	Post. edge of the sternocleidomastoid m.
V	Cranial edge of body of hyoid bone	CT slice encompassing the transverse cervical vessels[c]	Paraspinal (levator scapulae, splenius capitis) m.	Platysma m., skin	Post. edge of the sternocleidomastoid m.	Anterolateral border of the trapezius m.
VI	Caudal edge of body of thyroid cartilage[d]	Sternal manubrium	n.a.	Medial edges of thyroid gland, skin and anteromedial edge of sternocleidomastoid m.	Skin; platysma m.	Separation between trachea and esophagus[e]
RP	Base of skull	Cranial edge of the body of hyoid bone	Midline	Medial edge of int. carotid artery	Fascia under the pharyngeal mucosa	Prevertebral m. (longus colli, longus capitis)

[a] Midline structure lying between the medial borders of the anterior bellies of the digastric muscles
[b] The insertion of the thyroid muscle is often interposed between level Ia and the body of the hyoid bone
[c] For NPC, the reader is referred to the original description of the UICC/AJCC 1997 edition of the Ho's triangle. In essence, the fatty planes below and around the clavicle down to the trapezius muscle
[d] For paratracheal and recurrent nodes, the cranial border is the caudal edge of the cricoid cartilage
[e] For pretracheal nodes, trachea and anterior edge of cricoid cartilage

Source: Modified from Gregoire V, Levendag P, Ang KK, et al. (2003) [78]

Head and Neck Lymph Nodes

ANATOMICAL REFERENCE POINTS

1 – LONGUS CAPITIS MUSCLE
2 – INTERNAL CAROTID ARTERY
3 – STERNOCLEIDOMASTOID MUSCLE
4 – INTERNAL JUGULAR VEIN
5 – LATERAL PROCESS OF C1
6 – LONGUS COLLI MUSCLE
7 – GENIOGLOSSUS AND GENIOHYOID MUSCLES
8 – MYLOHYOID MUSCLE
9 – PARASPINAL (LEVATOR SCAPULAE) MUSCLE
10 – SUBMANDIBULAR GLAND
11 – ANTERIOR BELLY OF DIGASTRIC MUSCLE
12 – EXTERNAL CAROTID ARTERY
13 – POSTERIOR BELLY OF DIGASTRIC MUSCLE
14 – LEVATOR SCAPULAE MUSCLE
15 – SPLENIUS CAPITIS MUSCLE
16 – TRAPEZIUS MUSCLE
17 – HYOID BONE
18 – SCALENE MUSCLE
19 – COMMON CAROTID ARTERY
20 – CRICOID CARTILAGE
21 – THYROID CARTILAGE
22 – THYROID GLAND
23 – ANTERIOR SCALENE MUSCLE
24 – MIDDLE SCALENE MUSCLE
25 – POSTERIOR SCALENE MUSCLE
26 – TRANSVERSE CERVICAL VESSELS
27 – SUBCLAVIAN VEIN
28 – INNOMINATE VEIN

COLOR LEGEND

- LEVEL IA
- LEVEL IB
- LEVEL II
- LEVEL III
- LEVEL IV
- LEVEL V
- LEVEL VI
- RETROPHARYNGEAL NODES

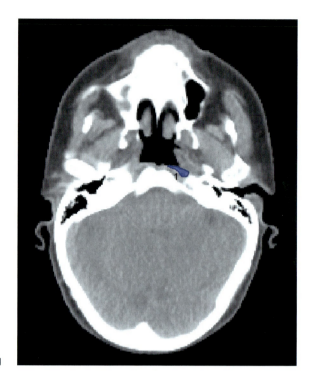

6.1

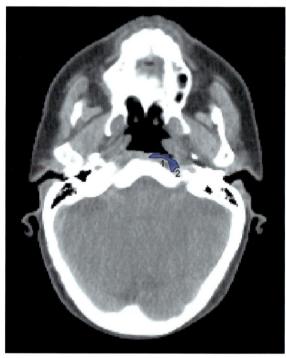

6.2

FIGS 6.1, 6.2

▬ RETROPHARYNGEAL NODES

1 – LONGUS CAPITIS MUSCLE
2 – INTERNAL CAROTID ARTERY

Head and Neck Lymph Nodes

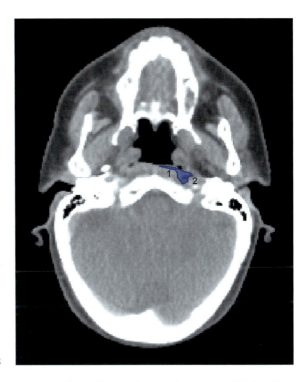

6.3

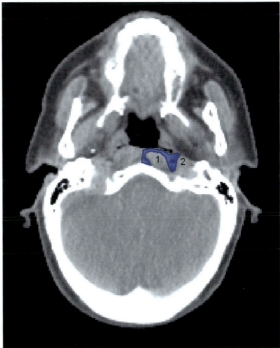

FIGS. 6.3, 6.4

- RETROPHARYNGEAL NODES

1 – LONGUS CAPITIS MUSCLE
2 – INTERNAL CAROTID ARTERY

6.4

A Guide for Delineation of Lymph Nodal Clinical Target Volume in Radiation Therapy

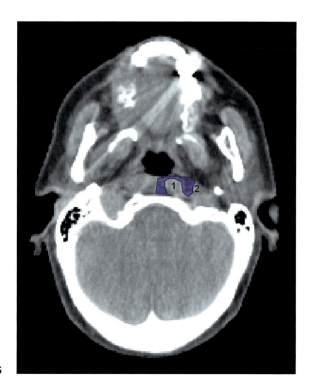

6.5

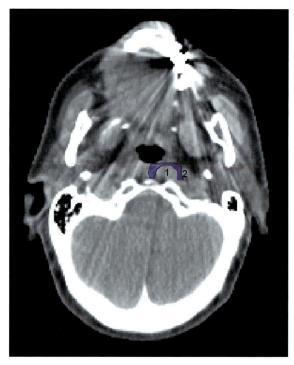

6.6

FIGS. 6.5, 6.6

▬ RETROPHARYNGEAL NODES

1 – LONGUS CAPITIS MUSCLE
2 – INTERNAL CAROTID ARTERY

Head and Neck Lymph Nodes

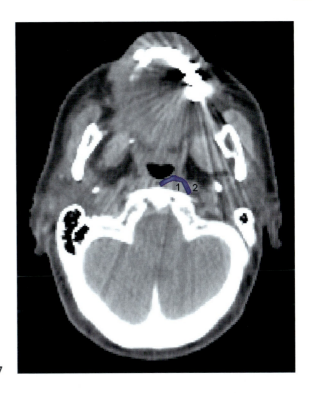

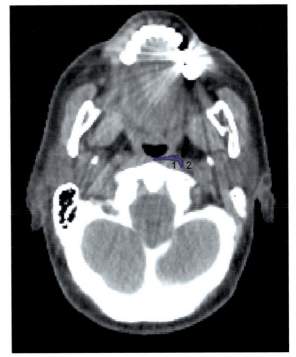

FIGS. 6.7, 6.8

- RETROPHARYNGEAL NODES

1 – LONGUS CAPITIS MUSCLE
2 – INTERNAL CAROTID ARTERY

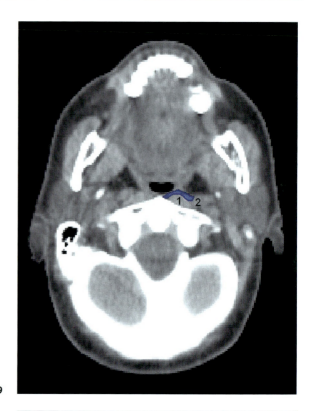

6.9

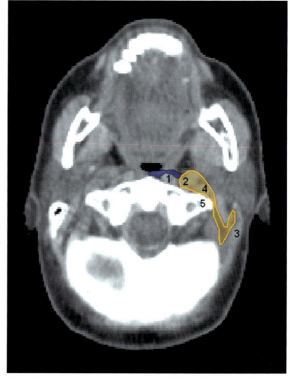

FIGS. 6.9, 6.10

- LEVEL II
- RETROPHARYNGEAL NODES

1 – LONGUS CAPITIS MUSCLE
2 – INTERNAL CAROTID ARTERY
3 – STERNOCLEIDOMASTOID MUSCLE
4 – INTERNAL JUGULAR VEIN
5 – LATERAL PROCESS OF C1

6.10

Head and Neck Lymph Nodes

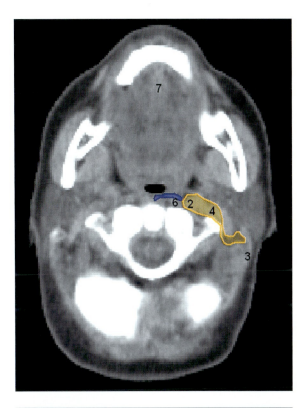

6.11

FIGS. 6.11, 6.12
- LEVEL II
- RETROPHARYNGEAL NODES

2 – INTERNAL CAROTID ARTERY
3 – STERNOCLEIDOMASTOID MUSCLE
4 – INTERNAL JUGULAR VEIN
6 – LONGUS COLLI MUSCLE
7 – GENIOGLOSSUS AND GENIOHYOID MUSCLES
8 – MYLOHYOID MUSCLE
9 – PARASPINAL (LEVATOR SCAPULAE) MUSCLE

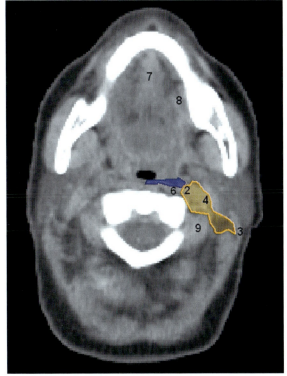

6.12

A Guide for Delineation of Lymph Nodal Clinical Target Volume in Radiation Therapy

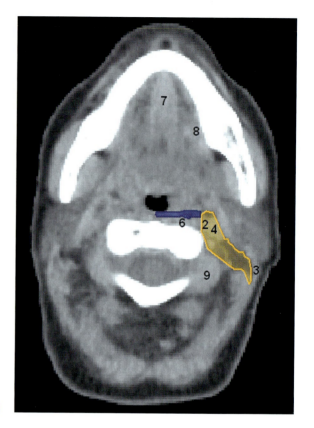

6.13

FIGS. 6.13, 6.14

- LEVEL IB
- LEVEL II
- RETROPHARYNGEAL NODES

2 – INTERNAL CAROTID ARTERY
3 – STERNOCLEIDOMASTOID MUSCLE
4 – INTERNAL JUGULAR VEIN
6 – LONGUS COLLI MUSCLE
7 – GENIOGLOSSUS AND GENIOHYOID MUSCLES
8 – MYLOHYOID MUSCLE
9 – PARASPINAL (LEVATOR SCAPULAE) MUSCLE
10 – SUBMANDIBULAR GLAND
11 – ANTERIOR BELLY OF DIGASTRIC MUSCLE

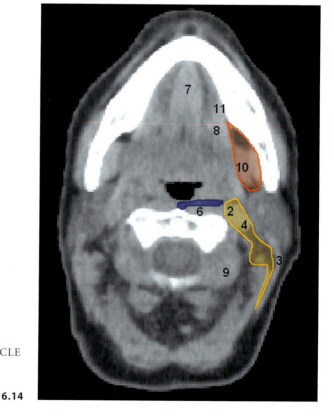

6.14

Head and Neck Lymph Nodes

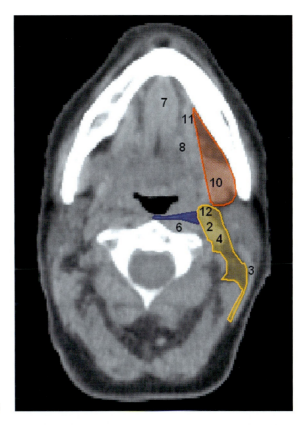

FIGS. 6.15, 6.16
- LEVEL IB
- LEVEL II
- RETROPHARYNGEAL NODES

2 – INTERNAL CAROTID ARTERY
3 – STERNOCLEIDOMASTOID MUSCLE
4 – INTERNAL JUGULAR VEIN
6 – LONGUS COLLI MUSCLE
7 – GENIOGLOSSUS AND GENIOHYOID MUSCLES
8 – MYLOHYOID MUSCLE
10 – SUBMANDIBULAR GLAND
11 – ANTERIOR BELLY OF DIGASTRIC MUSCLE
12 – EXTERNAL CAROTID ARTERY

A Guide for Delineation of Lymph Nodal Clinical Target Volume in Radiation Therapy

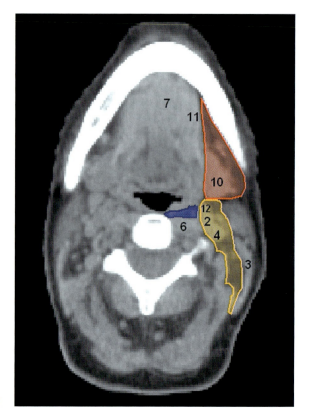

6.17

FIGS. 6.17, 6.18
- LEVEL IA
- LEVEL IB
- LEVEL II
- RETROPHARYNGEAL NODES

2 – INTERNAL CAROTID ARTERY
3 – STERNOCLEIDOMASTOID MUSCLE
4 – INTERNAL JUGULAR VEIN
6 – LONGUS COLLI MUSCLE
7 – GENIOGLOSSUS AND GENIOHYOID MUSCLES
10 – SUBMANDIBULAR GLAND
11 – ANTERIOR BELLY OF DIGASTRIC MUSCLE
12 – EXTERNAL CAROTID ARTERY
13 – POSTERIOR BELLY OF DIGASTRIC MUSCLE

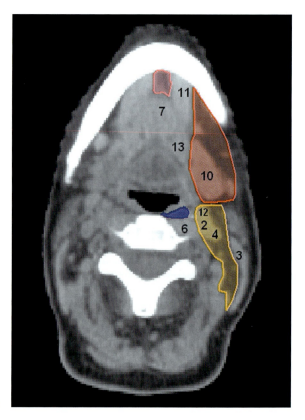

6.18

Head and Neck Lymph Nodes

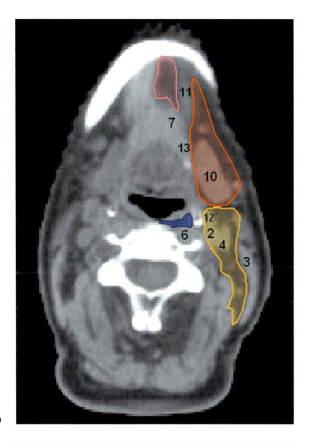

6.19

FIGS. 6.19, 6.20
- LEVEL IA
- LEVEL IB
- LEVEL II
- LEVEL V
- RETROPHARYNGEAL NODES

2 – INTERNAL CAROTID ARTERY
3 – STERNOCLEIDOMASTOID MUSCLE
4 – INTERNAL JUGULAR VEIN
6 – LONGUS COLLI MUSCLE
7 – GENIOHYOID MUSCLE
10 – SUBMANDIBULAR GLAND
11 – ANTERIOR BELLY OF DIGASTRIC MUSCLE
12 – EXTERNAL CAROTID ARTERY
13 – POSTERIOR BELLY OF DIGASTRIC MUSCLE
14 – LEVATOR SCAPULAE MUSCLE
15 – SPLENIUS CAPITIS MUSCLE
16 – TRAPEZIUS MUSCLE

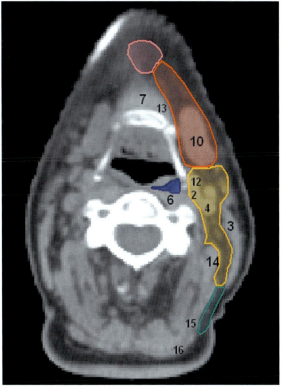

6.20

A Guide for Delineation of Lymph Nodal Clinical Target Volume in Radiation Therapy

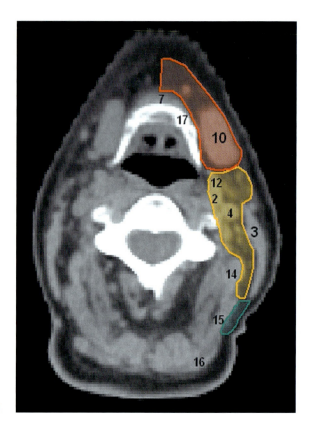

6.21

FIGS. 6.21, 6.22

- LEVEL IB
- LEVEL II
- LEVEL V

2 – INTERNAL CAROTID ARTERY
3 – STERNOCLEIDOMASTOID MUSCLE
4 – INTERNAL JUGULAR VEIN
7 – GENIOHYOID MUSCLE
10 – SUBMANDIBULAR GLAND
12 – EXTERNAL CAROTID ARTERY
14 – LEVATOR SCAPULAE MUSCLE
15 – SPLENIUS CAPITIS MUSCLE
16 – TRAPEZIUS MUSCLE
17 – HYOID BONE

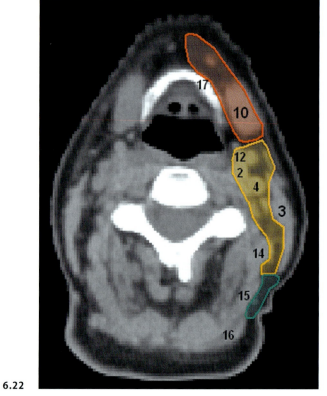

6.22

Head and Neck Lymph Nodes

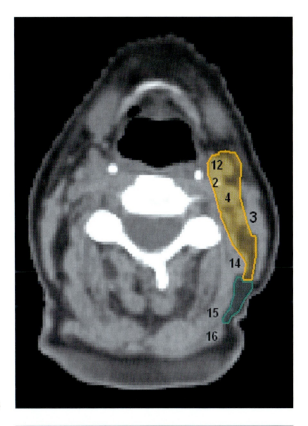

6.23

FIGS. 6.23, 6.24

- LEVEL II
- LEVEL III
- LEVEL V

2 – INTERNAL CAROTID ARTERY
3 – STERNOCLEIDOMASTOID MUSCLE
4 – INTERNAL JUGULAR VEIN
12 – EXTERNAL CAROTID ARTERY
14 – LEVATOR SCAPULAE MUSCLE
15 – SPLENIUS CAPITIS MUSCLE
16 – TRAPEZIUS MUSCLE
18 – SCALENE MUSCLE

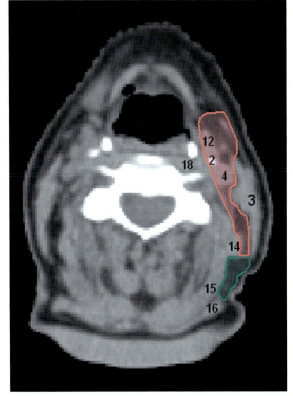

6.24

A Guide for Delineation of Lymph Nodal Clinical Target Volume in Radiation Therapy

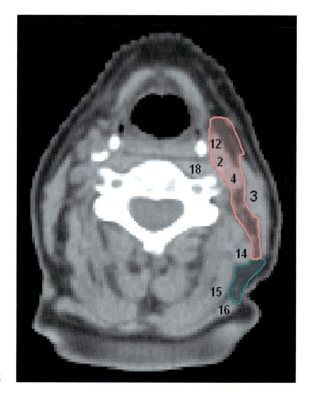

FIGS. 6.25, 6.26

- LEVEL III
- LEVEL V

 2 – INTERNAL CAROTID ARTERY
 3 – STERNOCLEIDOMASTOID MUSCLE
 4 – INTERNAL JUGULAR VEIN
12 – EXTERNAL CAROTID ARTERY
14 – LEVATOR SCAPULAE MUSCLE
15 – SPLENIUS CAPITIS MUSCLE
16 – TRAPEZIUS MUSCLE
18 – SCALENE MUSCLE

6.25

6.26

Head and Neck Lymph Nodes

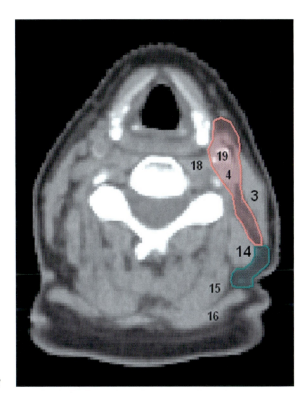

6.27

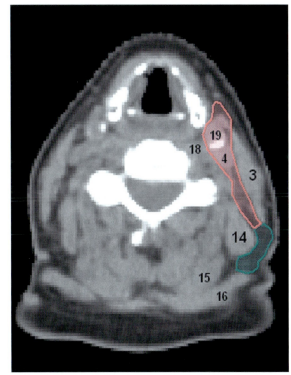

6.28

FIGS. 6.27, 6.28
- LEVEL III
- LEVEL V

 3 – STERNOCLEIDOMASTOID MUSCLE
 4 – INTERNAL JUGULAR VEIN
14 – LEVATOR SCAPULAE MUSCLE
15 – SPLENIUS CAPITIS MUSCLE
16 – TRAPEZIUS MUSCLE
18 – SCALENE MUSCLE
19 – COMMON CAROTID ARTERY

A Guide for Delineation of Lymph Nodal Clinical Target Volume in Radiation Therapy

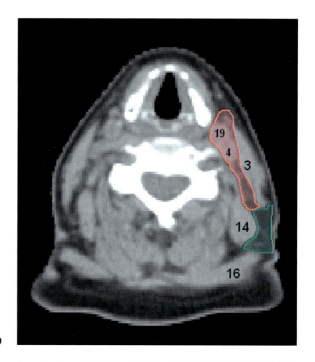

6.29

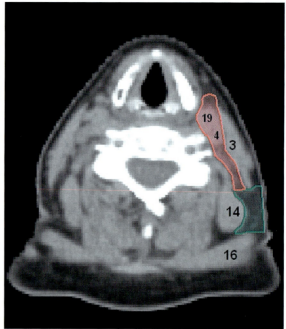

6.30

FIGS. 6.29, 6.30
- LEVEL III
- LEVEL V

3 – STERNOCLEIDOMASTOID MUSCLE
4 – INTERNAL JUGULAR VEIN
14 – LEVATOR SCAPULAE MUSCLE
16 – TRAPEZIUS MUSCLE
19 – COMMON CAROTID ARTERY

Head and Neck Lymph Nodes

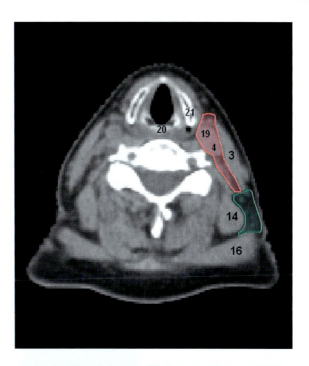

6.31

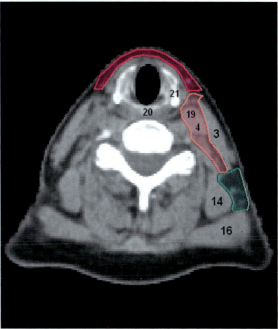

FIGS. 6.31, 6.32
- LEVEL III
- LEVEL V
- LEVEL VI

- 3 – STERNOCLEIDOMASTOID MUSCLE
- 4 – INTERNAL JUGULAR VEIN
- 14 – LEVATOR SCAPULAE MUSCLE
- 16 – TRAPEZIUS MUSCLE
- 19 – COMMON CAROTID ARTERY
- 20 – CRICOID CARTILAGE
- 21 – THYROID CARTILAGE

6.32

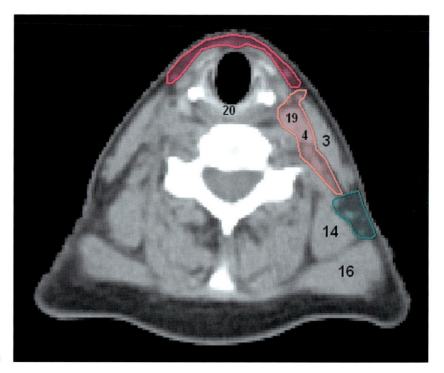

6.33

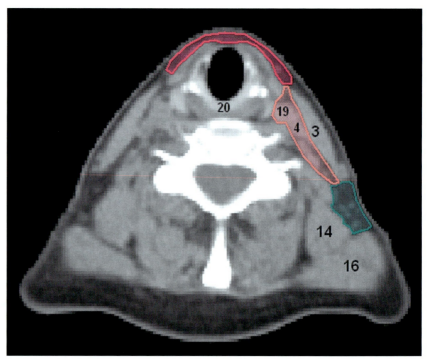

6.34

FIGS. 6.33, 6.34
- LEVEL III
- LEVEL V
- LEVEL VI

3 – STERNOCLEIDOMASTOID MUSCLE
4 – INTERNAL JUGULAR VEIN
14 – LEVATOR SCAPULAE MUSCLE
16 – TRAPEZIUS MUSCLE
19 – COMMON CAROTID ARTERY
20 – CRICOID CARTILAGE

Head and Neck Lymph Nodes

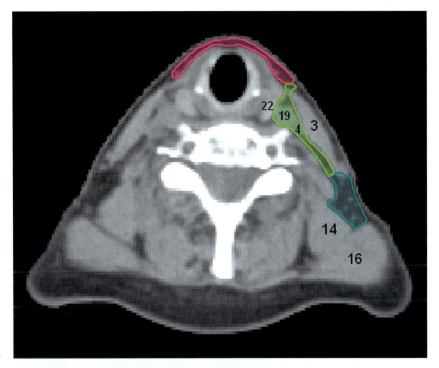

6.35

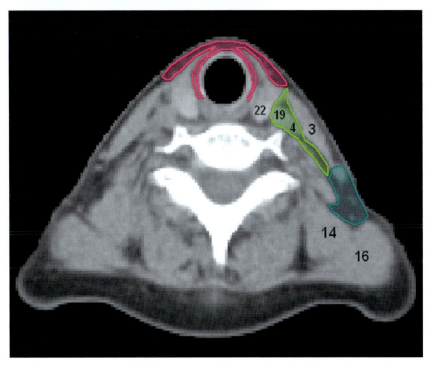

6.36

FIGS. 6.35, 6.36
- LEVEL IV
- LEVEL V
- LEVEL VI

3 – STERNOCLEIDOMASTOID MUSCLE
4 – INTERNAL JUGULAR VEIN
14 – LEVATOR SCAPULAE MUSCLE
16 – TRAPEZIUS MUSCLE
19 – COMMON CAROTID ARTERY
22 – THYROID GLAND

A Guide for Delineation of Lymph Nodal Clinical Target Volume in Radiation Therapy

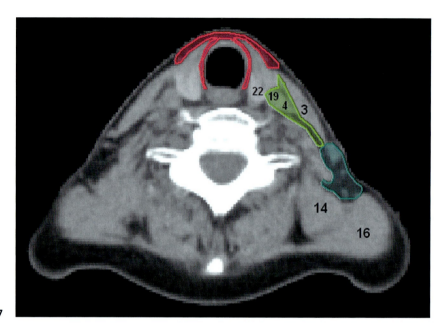

6.37

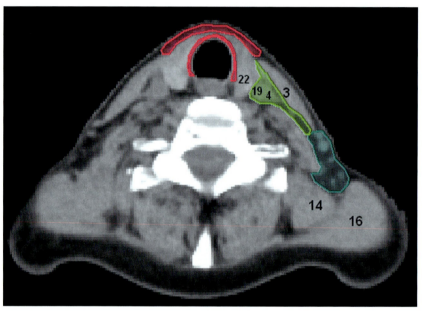

6.38

FIGS. 6.37, 6.38
- LEVEL IV
- LEVEL V
- LEVEL VI

3 – STERNOCLEIDOMASTOID MUSCLE
4 – INTERNAL JUGULAR VEIN
14 – LEVATOR SCAPULAE MUSCLE
16 – TRAPEZIUS MUSCLE
19 – COMMON CAROTID ARTERY
22 – THYROID GLAND

Head and Neck Lymph Nodes

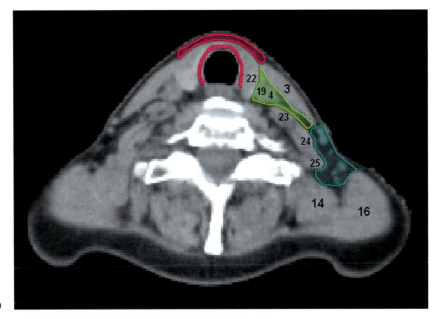

6.39

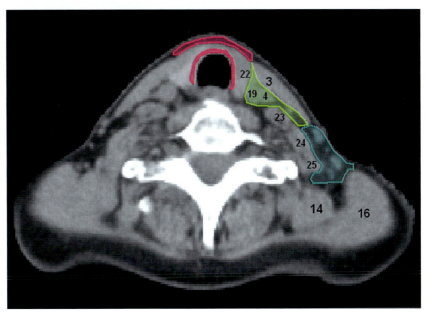

6.40

FIGS. 6.39, 6.40
- LEVEL IV
- LEVEL V
- LEVEL VI

3 – STERNOCLEIDOMASTOID MUSCLE
4 – INTERNAL JUGULAR VEIN
14 – LEVATOR SCAPULAE MUSCLE
16 – TRAPEZIUS MUSCLE
19 – COMMON CAROTID ARTERY
22 – THYROID GLAND
23 – ANTERIOR SCALENE MUSCLE
24 – MIDDLE SCALENE MUSCLE
25 – POSTERIOR SCALENE MUSCLE

A Guide for Delineation of Lymph Nodal Clinical Target Volume in Radiation Therapy

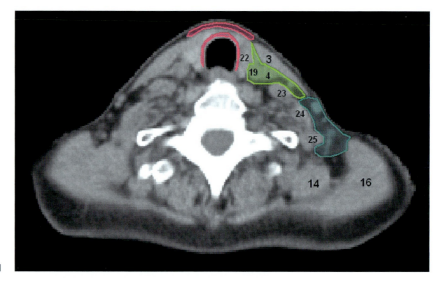

6.41

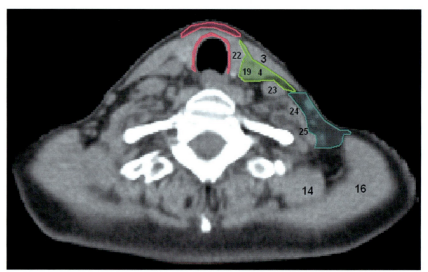

6.42

FIGS. 6.41, 6.42
- LEVEL IV
- LEVEL V
- LEVEL VI

3 – STERNOCLEIDOMASTOID MUSCLE
4 – INTERNAL JUGULAR VEIN
14 – LEVATOR SCAPULAE MUSCLE
16 – TRAPEZIUS MUSCLE
19 – COMMON CAROTID ARTERY
22 – THYROID GLAND
23 – ANTERIOR SCALENE MUSCLE
24 – MIDDLE SCALENE MUSCLE
25 – POSTERIOR SCALENE MUSCLE

Head and Neck Lymph Nodes

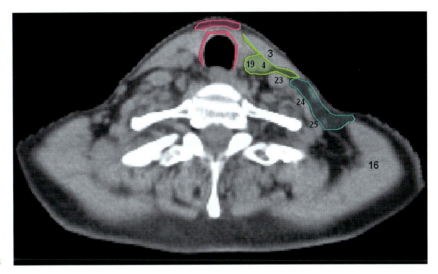

6.43

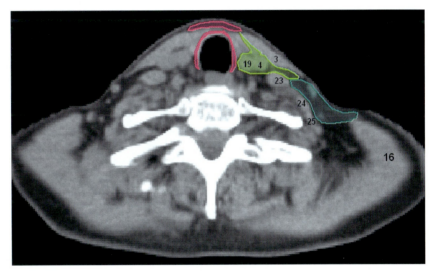

6.44

FIGS. 6.43, 6.44
- LEVEL IV
- LEVEL V
- LEVEL VI

3 – STERNOCLEIDOMASTOID MUSCLE
4 – INTERNAL JUGULAR VEIN
16 – TRAPEZIUS MUSCLE
19 – COMMON CAROTID ARTERY
23 – ANTERIOR SCALENE MUSCLE
24 – MIDDLE SCALENE MUSCLE
25 – POSTERIOR SCALENE MUSCLE

A Guide for Delineation of Lymph Nodal Clinical Target Volume in Radiation Therapy

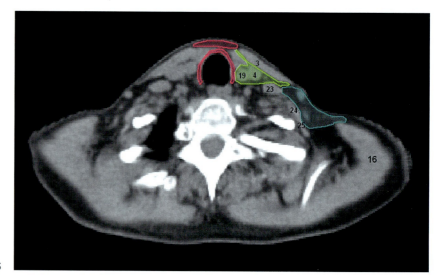

6.45

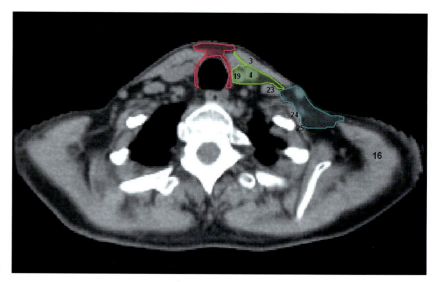

6.46

FIGS. 6.45, 6.46
- LEVEL IV
- LEVEL V
- LEVEL VI

3 – STERNOCLEIDOMASTOID MUSCLE
4 – INTERNAL JUGULAR VEIN
16 – TRAPEZIUS MUSCLE
19 – COMMON CAROTID ARTERY
23 – ANTERIOR SCALENE MUSCLE
24 – MIDDLE SCALENE MUSCLE
25 – POSTERIOR SCALENE MUSCLE

Head and Neck Lymph Nodes

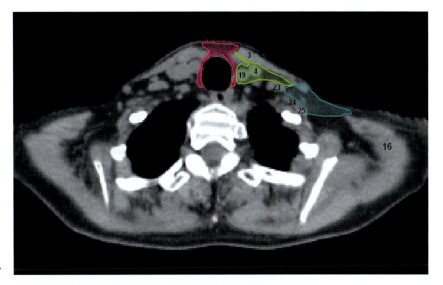

6.47

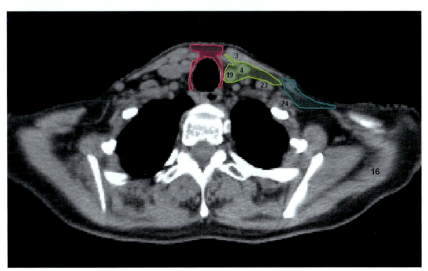

6.48

FIGS. 6.47, 6.48
- LEVEL IV
- LEVEL V
- LEVEL VI

3 – STERNOCLEIDOMASTOID MUSCLE
4 – INTERNAL JUGULAR VEIN
16 – TRAPEZIUS MUSCLE
19 – COMMON CAROTID ARTERY
23 – ANTERIOR SCALENE MUSCLE
24 – MIDDLE SCALENE MUSCLE
25 – POSTERIOR SCALENE MUSCLE

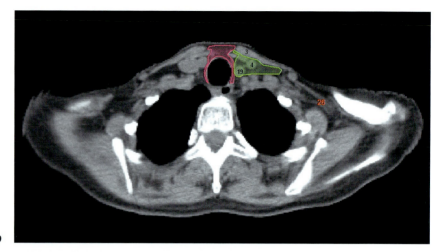

6.49

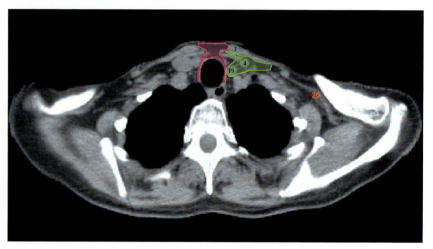

6.50

FIGS. 6.49, 6.50

- LEVEL IV
- LEVEL VI

3 – STERNOCLEIDOMASTOID MUSCLE
4 – INTERNAL JUGULAR VEIN
19 – COMMON CAROTID ARTERY
26 – TRANSVERSE CERVICAL VESSELS

Head and Neck Lymph Nodes

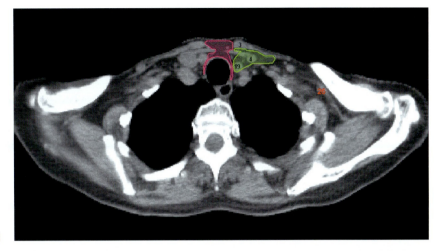

6.51

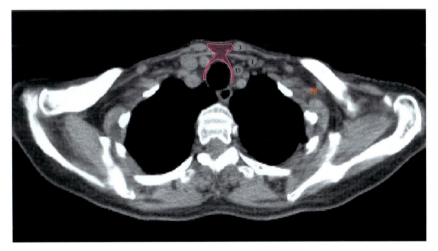

6.52

FIGS. 6.51, 6.52
- LEVEL IV
- LEVEL VI

3 – STERNOCLEIDOMASTOID MUSCLE
4 – INTERNAL JUGULAR VEIN
19 – COMMON CAROTID ARTERY
26 – TRANSVERSE CERVICAL VESSELS

A Guide for Delineation of Lymph Nodal Clinical Target Volume in Radiation Therapy

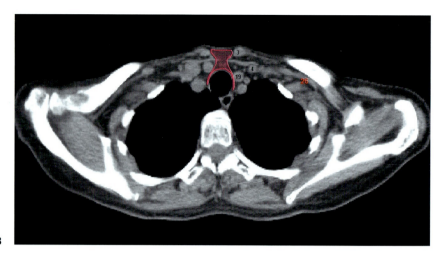

6.53

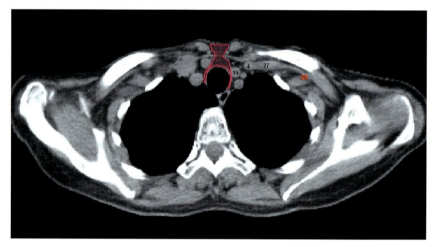

6.54

FIGS. 6.53, 6.54
— LEVEL VI

3 – STERNOCLEIDOMASTOID MUSCLE
4 – INTERNAL JUGULAR VEIN
19 – COMMON CAROTID ARTERY
26 – TRANSVERSE CERVICAL VESSELS
27 – SUBCLAVIAN VEIN

Head and Neck Lymph Nodes

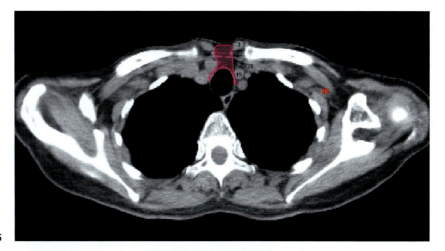

6.55

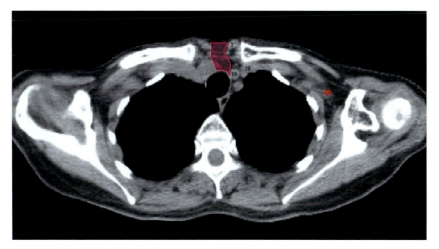

6.56

FIGS. 6.55, 6.56
— LEVEL VI

3 — STERNOCLEIDOMASTOID MUSCLE
19 — COMMON CAROTID ARTERY
26 — TRANSVERSE CERVICAL VESSELS
28 — INNOMINATE VEIN

A Guide for Delineation of Lymph Nodal Clinical Target Volume in Radiation Therapy

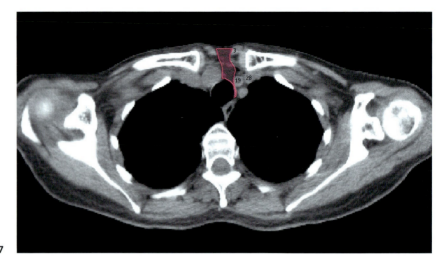

6.57

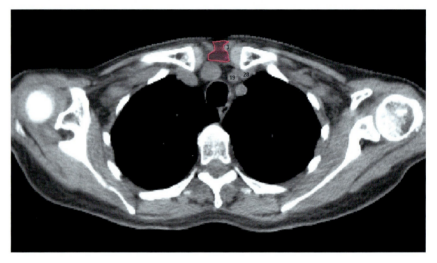

6.58

FIGS. 6.57, 6.58

■ LEVEL VI

3 – STERNOCLEIDOMASTOID MUSCLE
19 – COMMON CAROTID ARTERY
28 – INNOMINATE VEIN

Head and Neck Lymph Nodes

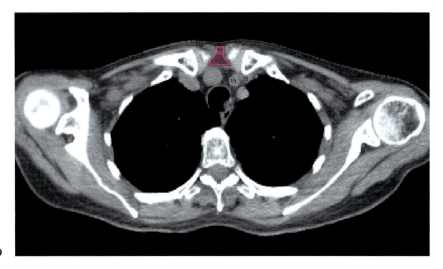

FIG. 6.59
— LEVEL VI

19 – COMMON CAROTID ARTERY
28 – INNOMINATE VEIN

Mediastinal Lymph Nodes

* This chapter has been written with the contributions
of Antonietta Augurio, Maria Luigia Storto, Maria Taraborrelli, and Lucia Anna Ursini

A Guide for Delineation of Lymph Nodal Clinical Target Volume in Radiation Therapy

SCOUT VIEW OF MEDIASTINUM

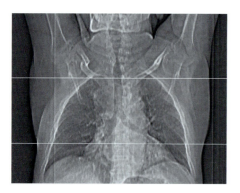

Station	Anatomical boundaries					
	Cranial	Caudal	Medial	Lateral	Anterior	Posterior
1R	Thoracic inlet[a]	Horizontal plane passing through line 1[b]	Trachea, thyroid	Right lung, right common carotid artery	Right clavicle, right brachiocephalic vein, thyroid	Anterior limit of station 3P, right subclavian artery
1L	Thoracic inlet[a]	Horizontal plane passing through line 1[b]	Trachea, thyroid	Left lung	Left subclavian vein, thyroid, left clavicle, left brachiocephalic vein	Anterior limit of station 3P, left subclavian artery, left common carotid artery
2R	Horizontal plane passing through line 1[b]	Horizontal plane passing through line 2[b]	Trachea, brachiocephalic trunk, station 2L	Right lung, right subclavian artery	Brachiocephalic trunk, right brachiocephalic vein, station 3A	Anterior limit of station 3P, trachea
2L	Horizontal plane passing through line 1[b]	Horizontal plane passing through line 2[b]	Trachea, station 2R	Left subclavian artery, left lung	Brachiocephalic trunk and left brachiocephalic vein	Anterior limit of station 3P, trachea
3A	Horizontal plane tangential to the top of sternal manubrium	Horizontal plane passing through line 2[b]	–	Right brachiocephalic vein, right and left lung	Sternum, clavicles	Thyroid, brachiocephalic trunk, right and left brachiocephalic veins
3P	Thoracic inlet[a]	Horizontal plane passing through carina	Esophagus	Right and left lung, right and left subclavian artery, descending aorta	Trachea, station 1R, station 1L, station 2R, station 2L, station 4R, station 4L	Esophagus, vertebral body
4R	Horizontal plane passing through line 2[b]	Horizontal plane passing through line 3[b]	Aortic arch, trachea, station 4L	Right lung, superior vena cava, arch of the azygos	Right brachiocephalic vein, aortic arch, ascending aorta	Right anterior-lateral wall of trachea, station 3P, right main bronchus
4L	Horizontal plane passing through line 2[b]	Horizontal plane passing through line 4[b]	Trachea, station 4R	Aortic arch, left pulmonary artery, ligamentum arteriosum	Ascending aorta, right and left pulmonary artery	Left anterior-lateral wall of the trachea, descending aorta, station 3P, left main bronchus
5	Horizontal plane passing through inferior border of aortic arch	Horizontal plane < through the most inferior aspect of left pulmonary artery	Ligamentum arteriosum, ascending aorta, main pulmonary artery	Left lung	Posterior limit of station 6	Descending aorta, left pulmonary artery
6	Horizontal plane passing through line 2[b]	Horizontal plane < through auricle of right atrium	–	Right and left lung	Sternum	Superior vena cava, left brachiocephalic vein, aortic arch, ascending aorta, pulmonary trunk, station 5
7	Horizontal plane extending across the carina	Horizontal plane passing through the most inferior aspect of right pulmonary artery (where the two main bronchi are neatly separated)	–	Medial wall of right and left main bronchi and of middle lobe bronchus	Right pulmonary artery	Esophagus, station 8
8	Inferior limit of station 3P	Diaphragm	–	Descending aorta, right lung, azygos vein	Left atrium, esophagus, station 7	Vertebral body

[a] The thoracic inlet marks the cervicothoracic junction. It can be represented by an imaginary plane tangential to the first rib and with oblique direction from the top downward and from the back toward the front
[b] For the definitions of the four main lines, see Chap. 3

Note: Hilar lymph nodes (stations 10R and 10L) lying adjacent to the bifurcation of the main bronchus in left and right lobar bronchi. The upper and lower limits are marked, respectively, by a plane cutting the main bronchi just below the carina and by a plane passing through the caudal limit of the main bronchi. These nodes are frequently located between the right and left pulmonary arteries and between the right and left main bronchi. Interlobar lymph nodes (stations 11R and 11L) are located in the fatty tissue lying between the lobar bronchi. The cranial limit of these nodal stations is therefore provided by the appearance of the lobar bronchi, while the caudal limit is provided by the further subdivision of the lobar bronchi on the axial plane. In the following images, stations 10 and 11 have been delineated as a single region

A Guide for Delineation of Lymph Nodal Clinical Target Volume in Radiation Therapy

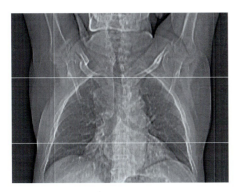

SCOUT VIEW OF MEDIASTINUM

Station	Anatomical boundaries					
	Cranial	Caudal	Medial	Lateral	Anterior	Posterior
1R	Thoracic inlet[a]	Horizontal plane passing through line 1[b]	Trachea, thyroid	Right lung, right common carotid artery	Right clavicle, right brachiocephalic vein, thyroid	Anterior limit of station 3P, right subclavian artery
1L	Thoracic inlet[a]	Horizontal plane passing through line 1[b]	Trachea, thyroid	Left lung	Left subclavian vein, thyroid, left clavicle, left brachiocephalic vein	Anterior limit of station 3P, left subclavian artery, left common carotid artery
2R	Horizontal plane passing through line 1[b]	Horizontal plane passing through line 2[b]	Trachea, brachiocephalic trunk, station 2L	Right lung, right subclavian artery	Brachiocephalic trunk, right brachiocephalic vein, station 3A	Anterior limit of station 3P, trachea
2L	Horizontal plane passing through line 1[b]	Horizontal plane passing through line 2[b]	Trachea, station 2R	Left subclavian artery, left lung	Brachiocephalic trunk and left brachiocephalic vein	Anterior limit of station 3P, trachea
3A	Horizontal plane tangential to the top of sternal manubrium	Horizontal plane passing through line 2[b]	–	Right brachiocephalic vein, right and left lung	Sternum, clavicles	Thyroid, brachiocephalic trunk, right and left brachiocephalic veins
3P	Thoracic inlet[a]	Horizontal plane passing through carina	Esophagus	Right and left lung, right and left subclavian artery, descending aorta	Trachea, station 1R, station 1L, station 2R, station 2L, station 4R, station 4L	Esophagus, vertebral body
4R	Horizontal plane passing through line 2[b]	Horizontal plane passing through line 3[b]	Aortic arch, trachea, station 4L	Right lung, superior vena cava, arch of the azygos	Right brachiocephalic vein, aortic arch, ascending aorta	Right anterior-lateral wall of trachea, station 3P, right main bronchus
4L	Horizontal plane passing through line 2[b]	Horizontal plane passing through line 4[b]	Trachea, station 4R	Aortic arch, left pulmonary artery, ligamentum arteriosum	Ascending aorta, right and left pulmonary artery	Left anterior-lateral wall of the trachea, descending aorta, station 3P, left main bronchus
5	Horizontal plane passing through inferior border of aortic arch	Horizontal plane < through the most inferior aspect of left pulmonary artery	Ligamentum arteriosum, ascending aorta, main pulmonary artery	Left lung	Posterior limit of station 6	Descending aorta, left pulmonary artery
6	Horizontal plane passing through line 2[b]	Horizontal plane < through auricle of right atrium	–	Right and left lung	Sternum	Superior vena cava, left brachiocephalic vein, aortic arch, ascending aorta, pulmonary trunk, station 5
7	Horizontal plane extending across the carina	Horizontal plane passing through the most inferior aspect of right pulmonary artery (where the two main bronchi are neatly separated)	–	Medial wall of right and left main bronchi and of middle lobe bronchus	Right pulmonary artery	Esophagus, station 8
8	Inferior limit of station 3P	Diaphragm	–	Descending aorta, right lung, azygos vein	Left atrium, esophagus, station 7	Vertebral body

[a] The thoracic inlet marks the cervicothoracic junction. It can be represented by an imaginary plane tangential to the first rib and with oblique direction from the top downward and from the back toward the front
[b] For the definitions of the four main lines, see Chap. 3

Note: Hilar lymph nodes (stations 10R and 10L) lying adjacent to the bifurcation of the main bronchus in left and right lobar bronchi. The upper and lower limits are marked, respectively, by a plane cutting the main bronchi just below the carina and by a plane passing through the caudal limit of the main bronchi. These nodes are frequently located between the right and left pulmonary arteries and between the right and left main bronchi. Interlobar lymph nodes (stations 11R and 11L) are located in the fatty tissue lying between the lobar bronchi. The cranial limit of these nodal stations is therefore provided by the appearance of the lobar bronchi, while the caudal limit is provided by the further subdivision of the lobar bronchi on the axial plane. In the following images, stations 10 and 11 have been delineated as a single region

Mediastinal Lymph Nodes

ANATOMICAL REFERENCE POINTS

1 – RIGHT SUBCLAVIAN VEIN
2 – RIGHT COMMON CAROTID ARTERY
3 – THYROID
4 – LEFT SUBCLAVIAN VEIN
5 – RIGHT SUBCLAVIAN ARTERY
6 – ESOPHAGUS
7 – LEFT COMMON CAROTID ARTERY
8 – LEFT SUBCLAVIAN ARTERY
9 – RIGHT BRACHIOCEPHALIC VEIN
10 – LEFT BRACHIOCEPHALIC VEIN
11 – BRACHIOCEPHALIC TRUNK
12 – AORTIC ARCH
13 – SUPERIOR VENA CAVA
14 – DESCENDING AORTA
15 – ASCENDING AORTA
16 – AZYGOS VEIN
17 – ARCH OF AZYGOS VEIN
18 – LEFT PULMONARY ARTERY
19 – MAIN PULMONARY ARTERY
20 – RIGHT PULMONARY ARTERY
21 – LEFT SUPERIOR PULMONARY VEIN
22 – RIGHT SUPERIOR PULMONARY VEIN
23 – RIGHT ATRIUM
24 – LEFT ATRIUM
25 – LEFT VENTRICLE

COLOR LEGEND

- HIGHEST MEDIASTINAL NODES (1)
- UPPER PARATRACHEAL NODES (2)
- PREVASCULAR (3A) AND RETROTRACHEAL NODES (3P)
- LOWER PARATRACHEAL NODES (4)
- SUBAORTIC NODES (5)
- PARA-AORTIC NODES (6)
- SUBCARINAL NODES (7)
- PARAESOPHAGEAL NODES (8)
- HILAR (10) AND INTERLOBAR (11) NODES

A Guide for Delineation of Lymph Nodal Clinical Target Volume in Radiation Therapy

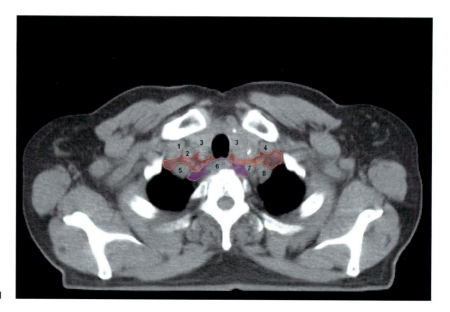

7.1

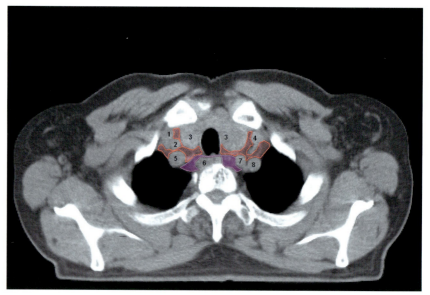

7.2

FIGS. 7.1, 7.2

- ▬ HIGHEST MEDIASTINAL NODES (1)
- ▬ PREVASCULAR (3A) AND RETROTRACHEAL NODES (3P)

1 – RIGHT SUBCLAVIAN VEIN
2 – RIGHT COMMON CAROTID ARTERY
3 – THYROID
4 – LEFT SUBCLAVIAN VEIN
5 – RIGHT SUBCLAVIAN ARTERY
6 – ESOPHAGUS
7 – LEFT COMMON CAROTID ARTERY
8 – LEFT SUBCLAVIAN ARTERY

Mediastinal Lymph Nodes 7

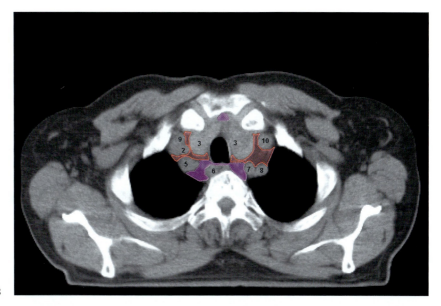

7.3

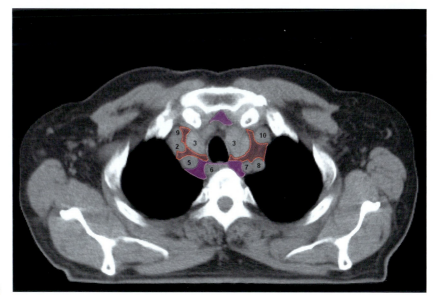

7.4

FIGS. 7.3, 7.4

- HIGHEST MEDIASTINAL NODES (1)
- PREVASCULAR (3A) AND RETROTRACHEAL NODES (3P)

2 – RIGHT COMMON CAROTID ARTERY
3 – THYROID
5 – RIGHT SUBCLAVIAN ARTERY
6 – ESOPHAGUS
7 – LEFT COMMON CAROTID ARTERY
8 – LEFT SUBCLAVIAN ARTERY
9 – RIGHT BRACHIOCEPHALIC VEIN
10 – LEFT BRACHIOCEPHALIC VEIN

A Guide for Delineation of Lymph Nodal Clinical Target Volume in Radiation Therapy

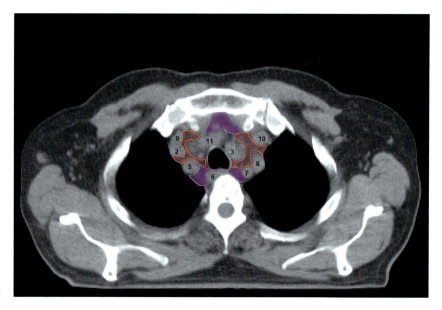

7.5

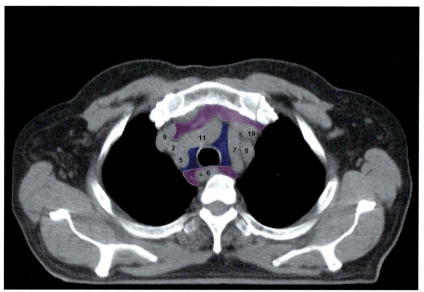

7.6

FIGS. 7.5, 7.6

- HIGHEST MEDIASTINAL NODES (1)
- UPPER PARATRACHEAL NODES (2)
- PREVASCULAR (3A) AND RETROTRACHEAL NODES (3P)

2 – RIGHT COMMON CAROTID ARTERY
3 – THYROID
5 – RIGHT SUBCLAVIAN ARTERY
6 – ESOPHAGUS
7 – LEFT COMMON CAROTID ARTERY
8 – LEFT SUBCLAVIAN ARTERY
9 – RIGHT BRACHIOCEPHALIC VEIN
10 – LEFT BRACHIOCEPHALIC VEIN
11 – BRACHIOCEPHALIC TRUNK

Mediastinal Lymph Nodes

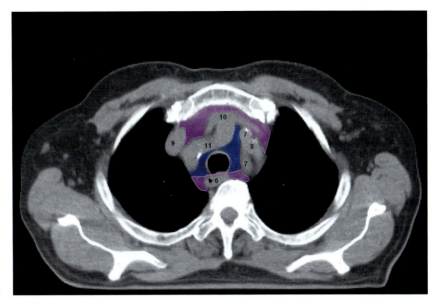

7.7

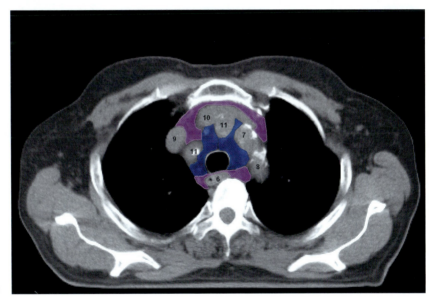

7.8

FIGS. 7.7, 7.8

- UPPER PARATRACHEAL NODES (2)
- PREVASCULAR (3A) AND RETROTRACHEAL NODES (3P)

6 – ESOPHAGUS
7 – LEFT COMMON CAROTID ARTERY
8 – LEFT SUBCLAVIAN ARTERY
9 – RIGHT BRACHIOCEPHALIC VEIN
10 – LEFT BRACHIOCEPHALIC VEIN
11 – BRACHIOCEPHALIC TRUNK

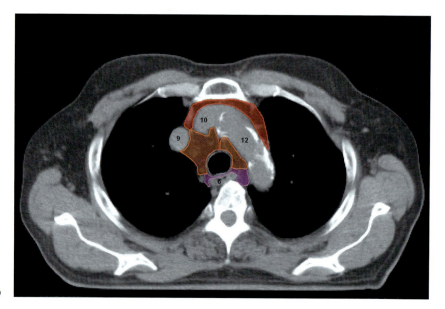

7.9

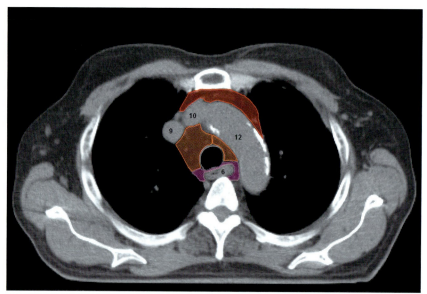

7.10

FIGS. 7.9, 7.10

- RETROTRACHEAL NODES (3P)
- LOWER PARATRACHEAL NODES (4)
- PARA-AORTIC NODES (6)

6 – ESOPHAGUS
9 – RIGHT BRACHIOCEPHALIC VEIN
10 – LEFT BRACHIOCEPHALIC VEIN
12 – AORTIC ARCH

Mediastinal Lymph Nodes

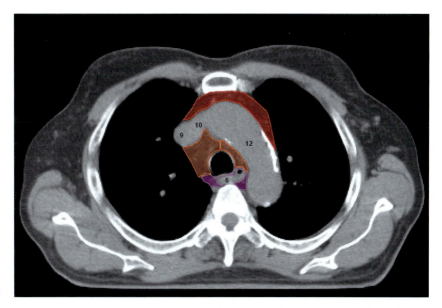

7.11

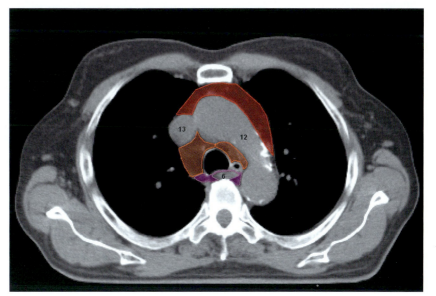

7.12

FIGS. 7.11, 7.12

- RETROTRACHEAL NODES (3P)
- LOWER PARATRACHEAL NODES (4)
- PARA-AORTIC NODES (6)

6 – ESOPHAGUS
9 – RIGHT BRACHIOCEPHALIC VEIN
10 – LEFT BRACHIOCEPHALIC VEIN
12 – AORTIC ARCH
13 – SUPERIOR VENA CAVA

A Guide for Delineation of Lymph Nodal Clinical Target Volume in Radiation Therapy

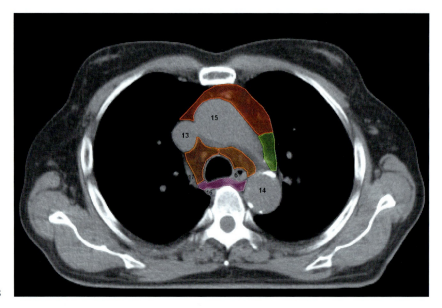

7.13

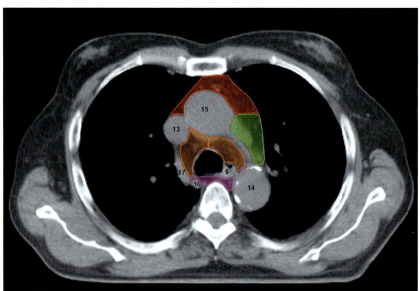

7.14

FIGS. 7.13, 7.14

- RETROTRACHEAL NODES (3P)
- LOWER PARATRACHEAL NODES (4)
- SUBAORTIC NODES (5)
- PARA-AORTIC NODES (6)

6 – ESOPHAGUS
13 – SUPERIOR VENA CAVA
14 – DESCENDING AORTA
15 – ASCENDING AORTA
16 – AZYGOS VEIN
17 – ARCH OF AZYGOS VEIN

Mediastinal Lymph Nodes

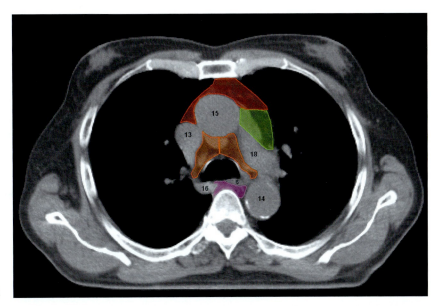

7.15

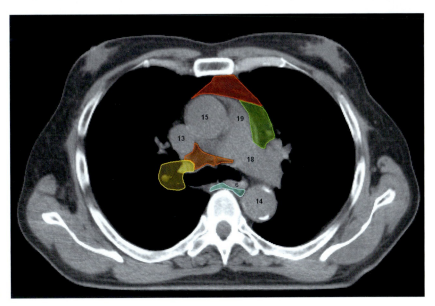

7.16

FIGS. 7.15, 7.16
- RETROTRACHEAL NODES (3P)
- LOWER PARATRACHEAL NODES (4)
- SUBAORTIC NODES (5)
- PARA-AORTIC NODES (6)
- PARAESOPHAGEAL NODES (8)
- HILAR (10) AND INTERLOBAR (11) NODES

6 – ESOPHAGUS
13 – SUPERIOR VENA CAVA
14 – DESCENDING AORTA
15 – ASCENDING AORTA
16 – AZYGOS VEIN
18 – LEFT PULMONARY ARTERY
19 – MAIN PULMONARY ARTERY

A Guide for Delineation of Lymph Nodal Clinical Target Volume in Radiation Therapy

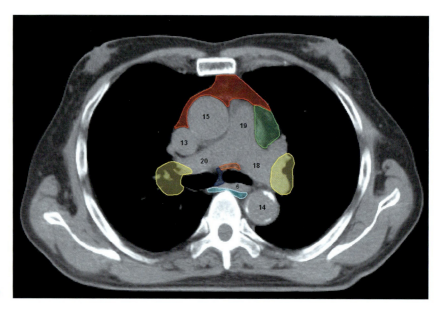

7.17

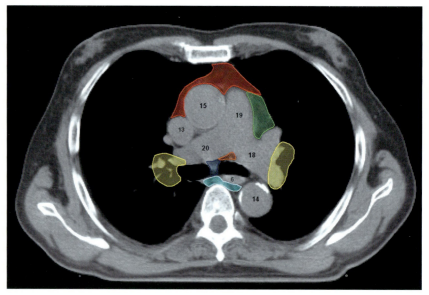

7.18

FIGS. 7.17, 7.18

- LOWER PARATRACHEAL NODES (4)
- SUBAORTIC NODES (5)
- PARA-AORTIC NODES (6)
- SUBCARINAL NODES (7)
- PARAESOPHAGEAL NODES (8)
- HILAR (10) AND INTERLOBAR (11) NODES

- 6 – ESOPHAGUS
- 13 – SUPERIOR VENA CAVA
- 14 – DESCENDING AORTA
- 15 – ASCENDING AORTA
- 18 – LEFT PULMONARY ARTERY
- 19 – MAIN PULMONARY ARTERY
- 20 – RIGHT PULMONARY ARTERY

Mediastinal Lymph Nodes

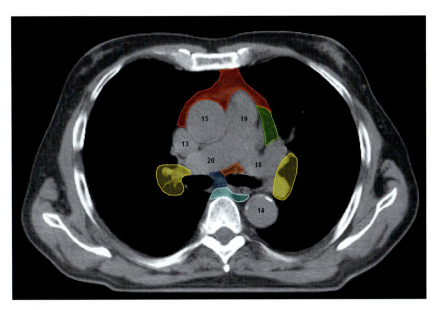

7.19

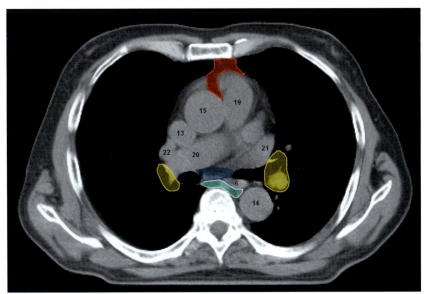

7.20

FIGS. 7.19, 7.20

- LOWER PARATRACHEAL NODES (4)
- SUBAORTIC NODES (5)
- PARA-AORTIC NODES (6)
- SUBCARINAL NODES (7)
- PARAESOPHAGEAL NODES (8)
- HILAR (10) AND INTERLOBAR (11) NODES

- 6 – ESOPHAGUS
- 13 – SUPERIOR VENA CAVA
- 14 – DESCENDING AORTA
- 15 – ASCENDING AORTA
- 18 – LEFT PULMONARY ARTERY
- 19 – MAIN PULMONARY ARTERY
- 20 – RIGHT PULMONARY ARTERY
- 21 – LEFT SUPERIOR PULMONARY VEIN
- 22 – RIGHT SUPERIOR PULMONARY VEIN

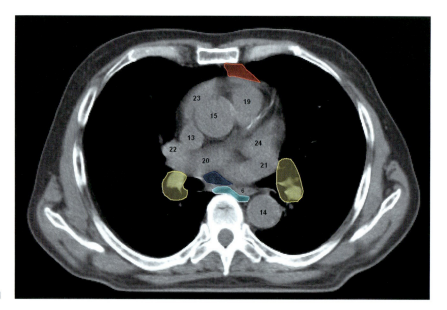

7.21

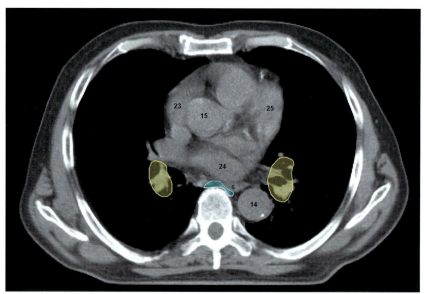

7.22

FIGS. 7.21, 7.22

- ▬ PARA-AORTIC NODES (6)
- ▬ SUBCARINAL NODES (7)
- ▬ PARAESOPHAGEAL NODES (8)
- ▬ HILAR (10) AND INTERLOBAR (11) NODES

- 6 – ESOPHAGUS
- 13 – SUPERIOR VENA CAVA
- 14 – DESCENDING AORTA
- 15 – ASCENDING AORTA
- 19 – MAIN PULMONARY ARTERY
- 20 – RIGHT PULMONARY ARTERY
- 21 – LEFT SUPERIOR PULMONARY VEIN
- 22 – RIGHT SUPERIOR PULMONARY VEIN
- 23 – RIGHT ATRIUM (AURICLE)
- 24 – LEFT ATRIUM (AURICLE)
- 25 – LEFT VENTRICLE

7 Mediastinal Lymph Nodes

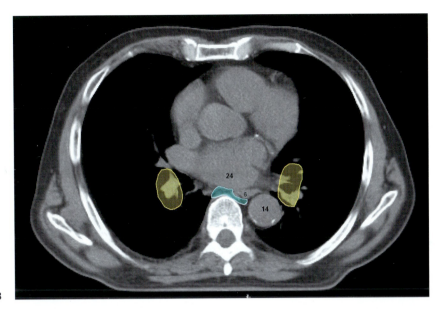

7.23

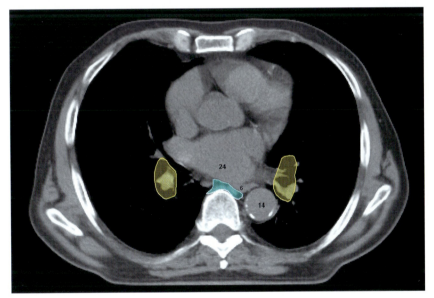

7.24

FIGS. 7.23, 7.24
- PARAESOPHAGEAL NODES (8)
- HILAR (10) AND INTERLOBAR (11) NODES

6 – ESOPHAGUS
14 – DESCENDING AORTA
24 – LEFT ATRIUM

A Guide for Delineation of Lymph Nodal Clinical Target Volume in Radiation Therapy

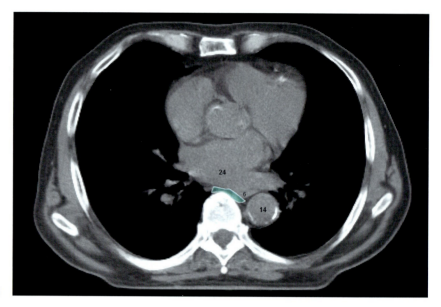

FIG. 7.25

▬ PARAESOPHAGEAL NODES (8)

6 – ESOPHAGUS
14 – DESCENDING AORTA
24 – LEFT ATRIUM

Upper Abdominal Region Lymph Nodes

* This chapter has been written with the contributions
of Antonietta Augurio, Raffaella Basilico, and Marco D'Alessandro

A Guide for Delineation of Lymph Nodal Clinical Target Volume in Radiation Therapy

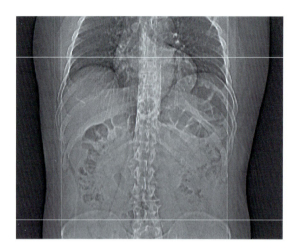

SCOUT VIEW OF
UPPER ABDOMINAL REGION

Station		Anatomical boundaries					
		Cranial	Caudal	Medial	Lateral	Anterior	Posterior
1	Right paracardial nodes	Plane through upper border of cardia (~T9–T10)	Plane through lower border of cardia (~T10–T11)	Cardia	Liver (superiorly), left diaphragmatic crus (inferiorly)	Liver	Cardia (superiorly), abdominal aorta (inferiorly)
2	Left paracardial nodes	Plane through upper border of cardia (~T9–T10)	Plane through lower border of cardia (~T10–T11)	Cardia	Stomach	Liver	Cardia (superiorly), abdominal aorta (inferiorly)
3	Nodes along the lesser curvature[a]	Plane through upper limit of the body and fundus of the stomach	Plane through lower limit of the body and fundus of the stomach	Left lobe of liver	Lesser gastric curvature	Fatty tissue	Stomach
7	Nodes along the left gastric artery						
4	Nodes along the greater gastric curvature	Plane through upper limit of the body and fundus of the stomach	Plane through lower limit of body of stomach	Greater gastric curvature	Intestine and left colic (splenic) flexure	Intestine	Spleen, anterior limit of station 10
5	Suprapyloric nodes	Plane through superior border of the pyloric region of the stomach	Plane through lower limit of the hepatic hilum	Fatty tissue	Ascending colon or liver (near the bed of the gallbladder)	Intestine	Pylorus
6	Infrapyloric nodes	Plane through upper limit of duodenum	1–1.5 cm caudal to the pylorus	Fatty tissue	Right colic (hepatic) flexure of the ascending colon or liver (near the bed of the gallbladder)	Intestine	Duodenum
8	Nodes along the common hepatic artery	Horizontal plane through the origin of celiac trunk	Intervertebral space T11–T12	Celiac trunk region (superiorly), pancreas (inferiorly)	Liver	Left lobe of liver (superiorly), antropyloric region (inferiorly)	Inferior vena cava
12	Nodes in the hepatoduodenal ligament						
9	Nodes around the celiac artery	Horizontal plane through the origin of celiac trunk	Plane passing above the origin of the mesenteric vessels	–	Liver (to the right), stomach (to the left)	Stomach	Aorta
10	Nodes at the splenic hilum	Superior limit of the vessels of splenic hilum	Lower limit of the vessels of splenic hilum	Body of stomach (superiorly), tail of pancreas (inferiorly)	Spleen	Posterior limit of station 4	Spleen
11	Nodes along the splenic artery	Superior limit of splenic artery	Lower limit of splenic artery	Abdominal aorta	Fatty tissue	Body of pancreas	Splenic hilum
13	Posterior pancreaticoduodenal nodes	Plane through superior border of the head of pancreas	Plane through lower border of the head of pancreas	Abdominal aorta	Descending (2nd) part of duodenum	Head of pancreas	Inferior vena cava
14	Nodes along the superior mesenteric vessels[b]	Superior limit of mesenteric vessels (~interspace T11–T12)	Plane through the origin of the superior mesenteric artery (~T12)	–	Head of pancreas	Head and isthmus of the pancreas	Abdominal aorta
16	Nodes around the abdominal aorta	Plane through upper limit of the celiac trunk	Aortic division into iliac vessels	–	–	–	Vertebral bodies
17	Anterior pancreaticoduodenal nodes	Plane through superior border of the head of pancreas	Plane through lower border of the head of pancreas	Intestine	Superior (1st) and descending (2nd) part of duodenum	Intestine	Head of pancreas
18	Nodes along the inferior margin of the pancreas	Plane through superior border of the body of pancreas	Caudal limit of the body and tail of pancreas	–	–	Head and tail of pancreas	Abdominal aorta, left kidney and left suprarenal gland
20	Nodes in the esophageal hiatus of the diaphragm	Carina	Esophageal hiatus of the diaphragm	–	Right: lung (superiorly), inferior vena cava (inferiorly) Left: left pulmonary hilum (superiorly), thoracic and abdominal aorta (inferiorly)	Bronchi (superiorly), heart and liver (inferiorly)	Vertebral bodies
110	Paraesophageal nodes in the lower thorax						
111	Supradiaphragmatic nodes						
112	Posterior mediastinal nodes						

[a] Station 19 (infradiaphragmatic lymph nodes) has been considered together with station 3 (lymph nodes along the lesser curvature)
[b] Station 15 (nodes along the middle colic vessels) has been considered together with station 14 (nodes along the superior mesenteric vessels)

A Guide for Delineation of Lymph Nodal Clinical Target Volume in Radiation Therapy

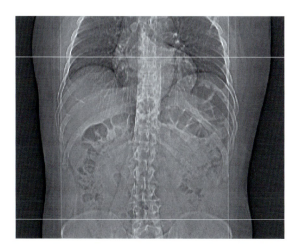

SCOUT VIEW OF UPPER ABDOMINAL REGION

Station		Anatomical boundaries					
		Cranial	Caudal	Medial	Lateral	Anterior	Posterior
1	Right paracardial nodes	Plane through upper border of cardia (~T9–T10)	Plane through lower border of cardia (~T10–T11)	Cardia	Liver (superiorly), left diaphragmatic crus (inferiorly)	Liver	Cardia (superiorly), abdominal aorta (inferiorly)
2	Left paracardial nodes	Plane through upper border of cardia (~T9–T10)	Plane through lower border of cardia (~T10–T11)	Cardia	Stomach	Liver	Cardia (superiorly), abdominal aorta (inferiorly)
3	Nodes along the lesser curvature[a]	Plane through upper limit of the body and fundus of the stomach	Plane through lower limit of the body and fundus of the stomach	Left lobe of liver	Lesser gastric curvature	Fatty tissue	Stomach
7	Nodes along the left gastric artery						
4	Nodes along the greater gastric curvature	Plane through upper limit of the body and fundus of the stomach	Plane through lower limit of body of stomach	Greater gastric curvature	Intestine and left colic (splenic) flexure	Intestine	Spleen, anterior limit of station 10
5	Suprapyloric nodes	Plane through superior border of the pyloric region of the stomach	Plane through lower limit of the hepatic hilum	Fatty tissue	Ascending colon or liver (near the bed of the gallbladder)	Intestine	Pylorus
6	Infrapyloric nodes	Plane through upper limit of duodenum	1–1.5 cm caudal to the pylorus	Fatty tissue	Right colic (hepatic) flexure of the ascending colon or liver (near the bed of the gallbladder)	Intestine	Duodenum
8	Nodes along the common hepatic artery	Horizontal plane through the origin of celiac trunk	Intervertebral space T11–T12	Celiac trunk region (superiorly), pancreas (inferiorly)	Liver	Left lobe of liver (superiorly), antropyloric region (inferiorly)	Inferior vena cava
12	Nodes in the hepatoduodenal ligament						
9	Nodes around the celiac artery	Horizontal plane through the origin of celiac trunk	Plane passing above the origin of the mesenteric vessels	–	Liver (to the right), stomach (to the left)	Stomach	Aorta
10	Nodes at the splenic hilum	Superior limit of the vessels of splenic hilum	Lower limit of the vessels of splenic hilum	Body of stomach (superiorly), tail of pancreas (inferiorly)	Spleen	Posterior limit of station 4	Spleen
11	Nodes along the splenic artery	Superior limit of splenic artery	Lower limit of splenic artery	Abdominal aorta	Fatty tissue	Body of pancreas	Splenic hilum
13	Posterior pancreaticoduodenal nodes	Plane through superior border of the head of pancreas	Plane through lower border of the head of pancreas	Abdominal aorta	Descending (2nd) part of duodenum	Head of pancreas	Inferior vena cava
14	Nodes along the superior mesenteric vessels[b]	Superior limit of mesenteric vessels (~interspace T11–T12)	Plane through the origin of the superior mesenteric artery (~T12)	–	Head of pancreas	Head and isthmus of the pancreas	Abdominal aorta
16	Nodes around the abdominal aorta	Plane through upper limit of the celiac trunk	Aortic division into iliac vessels	–	–	–	Vertebral bodies
17	Anterior pancreaticoduodenal nodes	Plane through superior border of the head of pancreas	Plane through lower border of the head of pancreas	Intestine	Superior (1st) and descending (2nd) part of duodenum	Intestine	Head of pancreas
18	Nodes along the inferior margin of the pancreas	Plane through superior border of the body of pancreas	Caudal limit of the body and tail of pancreas	–	–	Head and tail of pancreas	Abdominal aorta, left kidney and left suprarenal gland
20	Nodes in the esophageal hiatus of the diaphragm	Carina	Esophageal hiatus of the diaphragm	–	Right: lung (superiorly), inferior vena cava (inferiorly) Left: left pulmonary hilum (superiorly), thoracic and abdominal aorta (inferiorly)	Bronchi (superiorly), heart and liver (inferiorly)	Vertebral bodies
110	Paraesophageal nodes in the lower thorax						
111	Supradiaphragmatic nodes						
112	Posterior mediastinal nodes						

[a] Station 19 (infradiaphragmatic lymph nodes) has been considered together with station 3 (lymph nodes along the lesser curvature)
[b] Station 15 (nodes along the middle colic vessels) has been considered together with station 14 (nodes along the superior mesenteric vessels)

Upper Abdominal Region Lymph Nodes

ANATOMICAL REFERENCE POINTS

1 – DESCENDING AORTA
2 – ESOPHAGUS
3 – LIVER
4 – INFERIOR VENA CAVA
5 – LEFT DIAPHRAGMATIC CRUS
6 – SPLEEN
7 – STOMACH
8 – CARDIA
9 – 10TH THORACIC VERTEBRA
10 – VESSELS OF THE SPLENIC HILUM
11 – CELIAC TRUNK
12 – PYLORIC REGION OF THE STOMACH
13 – SPLENIC ARTERY
14 – PANCREAS
15 – 11TH THORACIC VERTEBRA
16 – GALLBLADDER
17 – HEPATIC FLEXURE OF THE ASCENDING COLON
18 – BODY OF PANCREAS
19 – TAIL OF PANCREAS
20 – DUODENUM
21 – ISTHMUS OF PANCREAS
22 – HEAD OF PANCREAS
23 – SUPERIOR MESENTERIC ARTERY
24 – ASCENDING COLON
25 – 12TH THORACIC VERTEBRA
26 – BIFURCATION OF THE ABDOMINAL AORTA

COLOR LEGEND

- RIGHT PARACARDIAL NODES (1)
- LEFT PARACARDIAL NODES (2)
- NODES ALONG LESSER GASTRIC CURVATURE (3) AND NODES ALONG THE LEFT GASTRIC ARTERY (7)
- NODES ALONG THE GREATER GASTRIC CURVATURE (4)
- SUPRAPYLORIC NODES (5)
- INFRAPYLORIC NODES (6)
- NODES ALONG THE COMMON HEPATIC ARTERY (8) AND NODES IN THE HEPATODUODENAL LIGAMENT (12)
- CELIAC NODES (9)
- NODES AT THE SPLENIC HILUM (10)
- NODES ALONG THE SPLENIC ARTERY (11)
- POSTERIOR PANCREATICODUODENAL NODES (13)
- NODES ALONG THE SUPERIOR MESENTERIC VESSELS (14)
- NODES AROUND THE ABDOMINAL AORTA (16)
- ANTERIOR PANCREATICODUODENAL NODES (17)
- NODES ALONG THE INFERIOR MARGIN OF THE PANCREAS (18)
- PERIESOPHAGEAL NODES: NODES IN THE ESOPHAGEAL HIATUS OF THE DIAPHRAGM (20), PARAESOPHAGEAL NODES IN THE LOWER THORAX (110), SUPRADIAPHRAGMATIC NODES (111), AND POSTERIOR MEDIASTINAL NODES (112)

A Guide for Delineation of Lymph Nodal Clinical Target Volume in Radiation Therapy

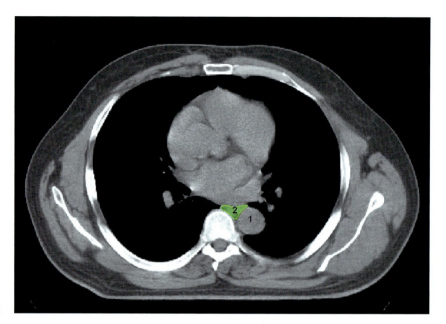

8.1

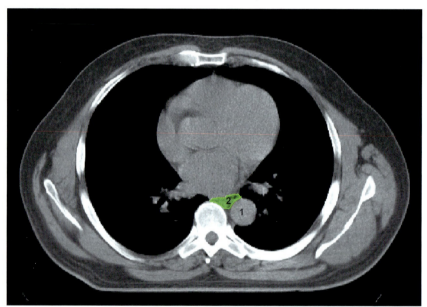

8.2

FIGS. 8.1, 8.2

- PERIESOPHAGEAL NODES: NODES IN THE ESOPHAGEAL HIATUS OF THE DIAPHRAGM (20), PARAESOPHAGEAL NODES IN THE LOWER THORAX (110), SUPRADIAPHRAGMATIC NODES (111) AND POSTERIOR MEDIASTINAL NODES (112)

1 – DESCENDING AORTA
2 – ESOPHAGUS

Upper Abdominal Region Lymph Nodes

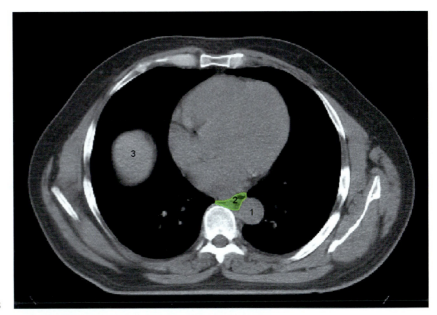

8.3

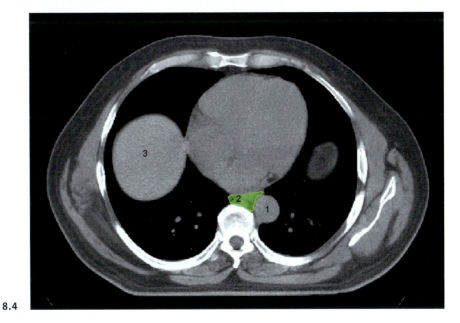

8.4

FIGS. 8.3, 8.4

- PERIESOPHAGEAL NODES: NODES IN THE ESOPHAGEAL HIATUS OF THE DIAPHRAGM (20), PARAESOPHAGEAL NODES IN THE LOWER THORAX (110), SUPRADIAPHRAGMATIC NODES (111) AND POSTERIOR MEDIASTINAL NODES (112)

1 – DESCENDING AORTA
2 – ESOPHAGUS
3 – LIVER

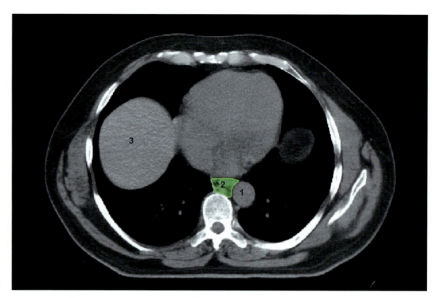

8.5

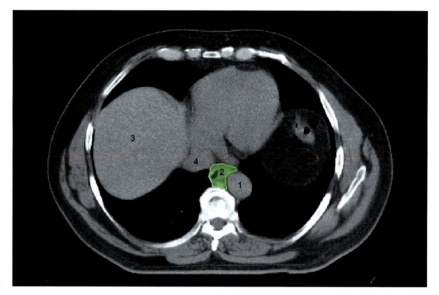

8.6

FIGS. 8.5, 8.6

▬ PERIESOPHAGEAL NODES: NODES IN THE ESOPHAGEAL HIATUS OF THE DIAPHRAGM (20), PARAESOPHAGEAL NODES IN THE LOWER THORAX (110), SUPRADIAPHRAGMATIC NODES (111) AND POSTERIOR MEDIASTINAL NODES (112)

1 – DESCENDING AORTA
2 – ESOPHAGUS
3 – LIVER
4 – INFERIOR VENA CAVA

Upper Abdominal Region Lymph Nodes

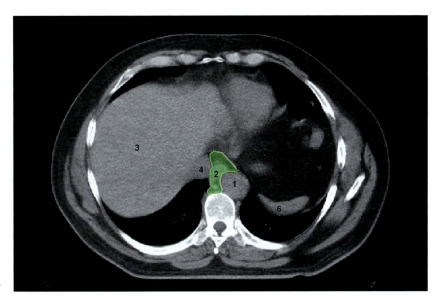

8.7

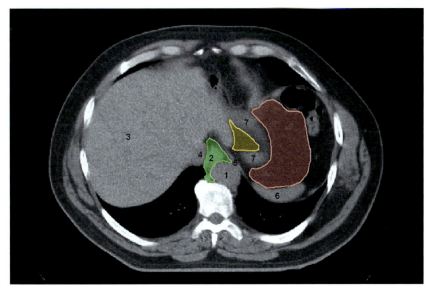

8.8

FIGS. 8.7, 8.8

- NODES ALONG THE LESSER GASTRIC CURVATURE (3) AND NODES ALONG THE LEFT GASTRIC ARTERY (7)
- NODES ALONG THE GREATER GASTRIC CURVATURE (4)
- PERIESOPHAGEAL NODES: NODES IN THE ESOPHAGEAL HIATUS OF THE DIAPHRAGM (20), PARAESOPHAGEAL NODES IN THE LOWER THORAX (110), SUPRADIAPHRAGMATIC NODES (111) AND POSTERIOR MEDIASTINAL NODES (112)

1 – DESCENDING AORTA
2 – ESOPHAGUS
3 – LIVER
4 – INFERIOR VENA CAVA
5 – LEFT DIAPHRAGMATIC CRUS
6 – SPLEEN
7 – STOMACH

A Guide for Delineation of Lymph Nodal Clinical Target Volume in Radiation Therapy

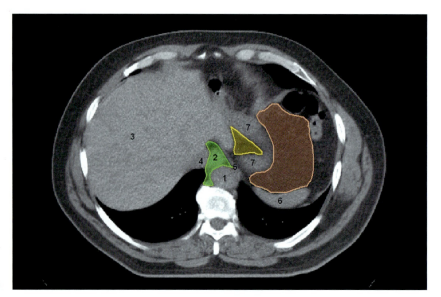

8.9

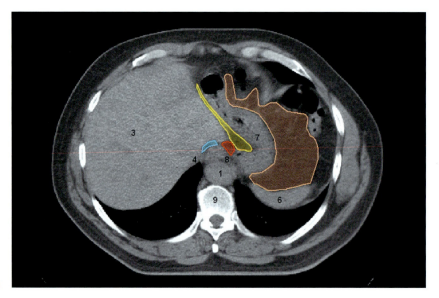

8.10

FIGS. 8.9, 8.10

- RIGHT PARACARDIAL NODES (1)
- LEFT PARACARDIAL NODES (2)
- NODES ALONG THE LESSER GASTRIC CURVATURE (3) AND NODES ALONG THE LEFT GASTRIC ARTERY (7)
- NODES ALONG THE GREATER GASTRIC CURVATURE (4)
- PERIESOPHAGEAL NODES: NODES IN THE ESOPHAGEAL HIATUS OF THE DIAPHRAGM (20), PARAESOPHAGEAL NODES IN THE LOWER THORAX (110), SUPRADIAPHRAGMATIC NODES (111) AND POSTERIOR MEDIASTINAL NODES (112)

1 – DESCENDING AORTA
2 – ESOPHAGUS
3 – LIVER
4 – INFERIOR VENA CAVA
5 – LEFT DIAPHRAGMATIC CRUS
6 – SPLEEN
7 – STOMACH
8 – CARDIA
9 – 10TH THORACIC VERTEBRA

Upper Abdominal Region Lymph Nodes

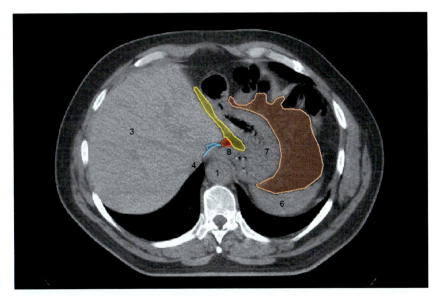

8.11

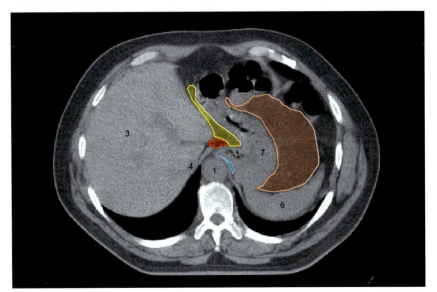

8.12

FIGS. 8.11, 8.12

- RIGHT PARACARDIAL NODES (1)
- LEFT PARACARDIAL NODES (2)
- NODES ALONG THE LESSER GASTRIC CURVATURE (3) AND NODES ALONG THE LEFT GASTRIC ARTERY (7)
- NODES ALONG THE GREATER GASTRIC CURVATURE (4)

1 – DESCENDING AORTA
3 – LIVER
4 – INFERIOR VENA CAVA
6 – SPLEEN
7 – STOMACH
8 – CARDIA

A Guide for Delineation of Lymph Nodal Clinical Target Volume in Radiation Therapy

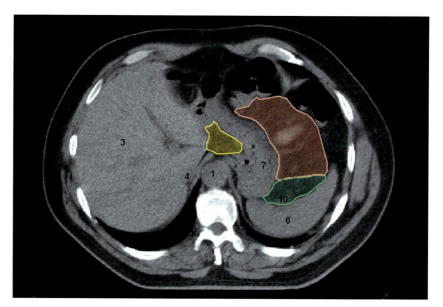

8.13

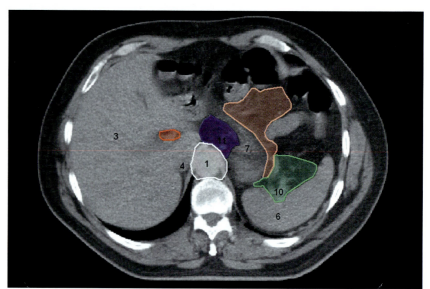

8.14

FIGS. 8.13, 8.14

- NODES ALONG THE LESSER GASTRIC CURVATURE (3) AND NODES ALONG THE LEFT GASTRIC ARTERY (7)
- NODES ALONG THE GREATER GASTRIC CURVATURE (4)
- NODES ALONG THE COMMON HEPATIC ARTERY (8) AND NODES IN THE HEPATODUODENAL LIGAMENT (12)
- CELIAC NODES (9).
- NODES AT THE SPLENIC HILUM (10)
- NODES AROUND THE ABDOMINAL AORTA (16)

1 – DESCENDING AORTA
3 – LIVER
4 – INFERIOR VENA CAVA
6 – SPLEEN
7 – STOMACH
10 – VESSELS OF THE SPLENIC HILUM
11 – CELIAC TRUNK

Upper Abdominal Region Lymph Nodes

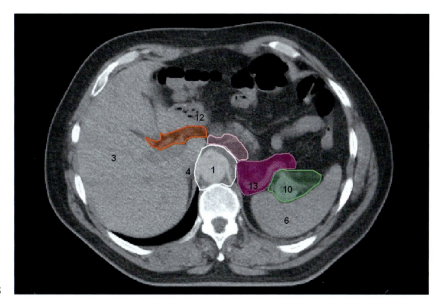

8.15

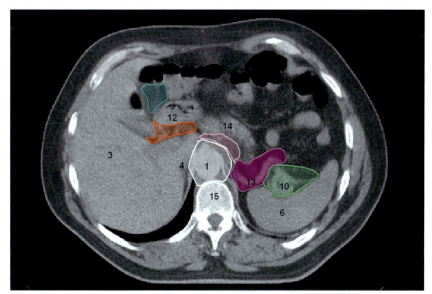

8.16

FIGS. 8.15, 8.16

- SUPRAPYLORIC NODES (5)
- NODES ALONG THE COMMON HEPATIC ARTERY (8) AND NODES IN THE HEPATODUO-DENAL LIGAMENT (12)
- NODES AT THE SPLENIC HILUM (10)
- NODES ALONG THE SPLENIC ARTERY (11)
- NODES AROUND THE ABDOMINAL AORTA (16)
- NODES ALONG THE INFERIOR MARGIN OF THE PANCREAS (18)

1 – DESCENDING AORTA
3 – LIVER
4 – INFERIOR VENA CAVA
6 – SPLEEN
10 – VESSELS OF THE SPLENIC HILUM
12 – PYLORIC REGION OF THE STOMACH
13 – SPLENIC ARTERY
14 – PANCREAS
15 – 11TH THORACIC VERTEBRA

A Guide for Delineation of Lymph Nodal Clinical Target Volume in Radiation Therapy

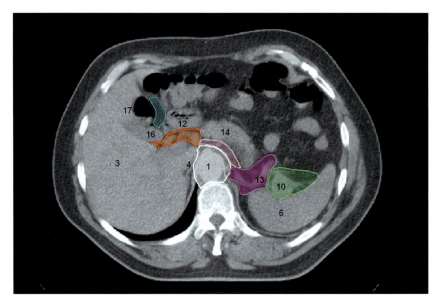

8.17

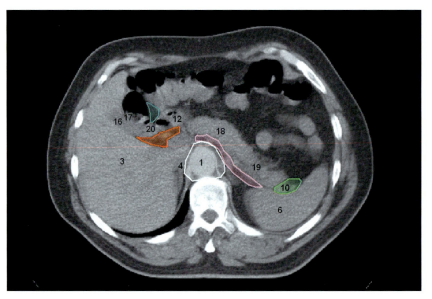

8.18

FIGS. 8.17, 8.18

- SUPRAPYLORIC NODES (5)
- NODES ALONG THE COMMON HEPATIC ARTERY (8) AND NODES IN THE HEPATODUODENAL LIGAMENT (12)
- NODES AT THE SPLENIC HILUM (10)
- NODES ALONG THE SPLENIC ARTERY (11)
- NODES AROUND THE ABDOMINAL AORTA (16).
- NODES ALONG THE INFERIOR MARGIN OF THE PANCREAS (18)

1 – DESCENDING AORTA
3 – LIVER
4 – INFERIOR VENA CAVA
6 – SPLEEN
10 – VESSELS OF THE SPLENIC HILUM
12 – PYLORIC REGION OF THE STOMACH
13 – SPLENIC ARTERY
14 – PANCREAS
16 – GALLBLADDER
17 – HEPATIC FLEXURE OF THE ASCENDING COLON
18 – BODY OF PANCREAS
19 – TAIL OF PANCREAS
20 – DUODENUM

Upper Abdominal Region Lymph Nodes

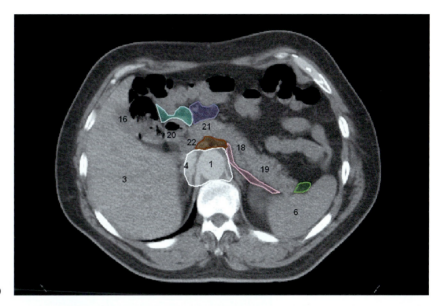

8.19

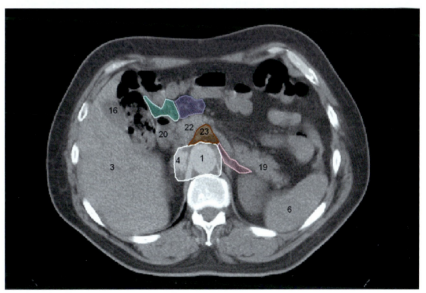

8.20

FIGS. 8.19, 8.20

- INFRAPYLORIC NODES (6)
- NODES AT THE SPLENIC HILUM (10)
- NODES ALONG THE SUPERIOR MESENTERIC VESSELS (14)
- NODES AROUND THE ABDOMINAL AORTA (16)
- ANTERIOR PANCREATICODUODENAL NODES (17)
- NODES ALONG THE INFERIOR MARGIN OF THE PANCREAS (18)

1 – DESCENDING AORTA
3 – LIVER
4 – INFERIOR VENA CAVA
6 – SPLEEN
16 – GALLBLADDER
18 – BODY OF PANCREAS
19 – TAIL OF PANCREAS
20 – DUODENUM
21 – ISTHMUS OF PANCREAS
22 – HEAD OF PANCREAS
23 – SUPERIOR MESENTERIC ARTERY

A Guide for Delineation of Lymph Nodal Clinical Target Volume in Radiation Therapy

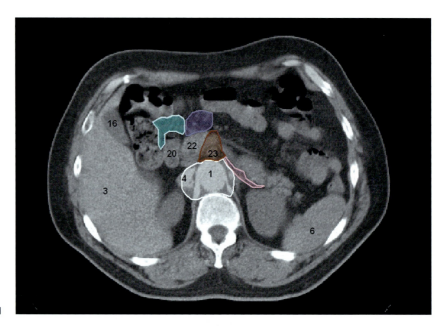

8.21

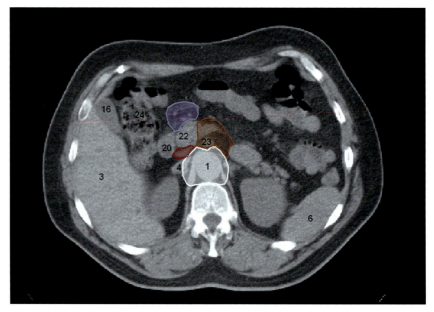

8.22

FIGS. 8.21, 8.22

- INFRAPYLORIC NODES (6)
- POSTERIOR PANCREATICODUODENAL NODES (13)
- NODES ALONG THE SUPERIOR MESENTERIC VESSELS (14)
- NODES AROUND THE ABDOMINAL AORTA (16)
- ANTERIOR PANCREATICODUODENAL NODES (17)
- NODES ALONG THE INFERIOR MARGIN OF THE PANCREAS (18).

1 – DESCENDING AORTA
3 – LIVER
4 – INFERIOR VENA CAVA
6 – SPLEEN
16 – GALLBLADDER
20 – DUODENUM
22 – HEAD OF PANCREAS
23 – SUPERIOR MESENTERIC ARTERY
24 – ASCENDING COLON

Upper Abdominal Region Lymph Nodes

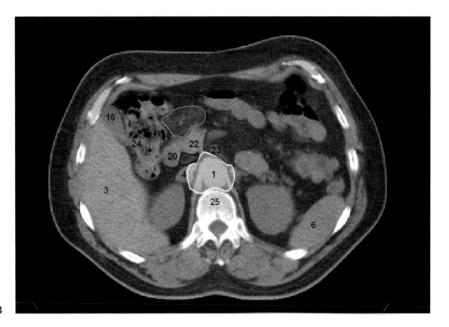

8.23

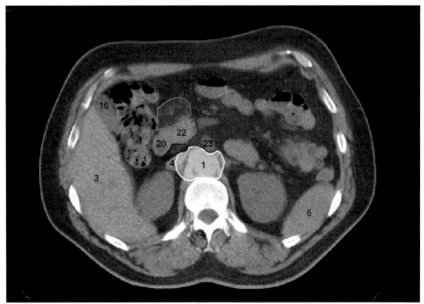

8.24

FIGS. 8.23, 8.24

- POSTERIOR PANCREATICODUODENAL NODES (13)
- NODES ALONG THE SUPERIOR MESENTERIC VESSELS (14)
- NODES AROUND THE ABDOMINAL AORTA (16)
- ANTERIOR PANCREATICODUODENAL NODES (17)

1 – DESCENDING AORTA
3 – LIVER
4 – INFERIOR VENA CAVA
6 – SPLEEN
16 – GALLBLADDER
20 – DUODENUM
22 – HEAD OF PANCREAS
23 – SUPERIOR MESENTERIC ARTERY
24 – ASCENDING COLON
25 – 12TH THORACIC VERTEBRA

A Guide for Delineation of Lymph Nodal Clinical Target Volume in Radiation Therapy

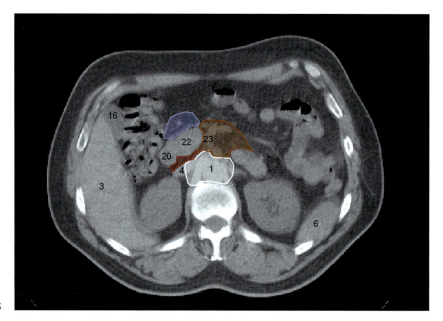

8.25

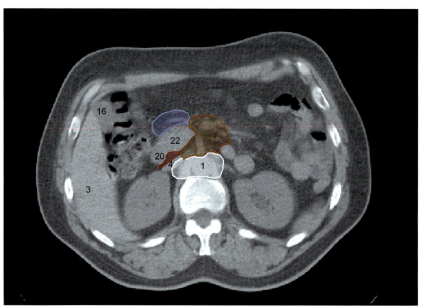

8.26

FIGS. 8.25, 8.26

- POSTERIOR PANCREATICODUODENAL NODES (13)
- NODES ALONG THE SUPERIOR MESENTERIC VESSELS (14)
- NODES AROUND THE ABDOMINAL AORTA (16)
- ANTERIOR PANCREATICODUODENAL NODES (17)

1 – DESCENDING AORTA
3 – LIVER
4 – INFERIOR VENA CAVA
6 – SPLEEN
16 – GALLBLADDER
20 – DUODENUM
22 – HEAD OF PANCREAS
23 – SUPERIOR MESENTERIC ARTERY

Upper Abdominal Region Lymph Nodes

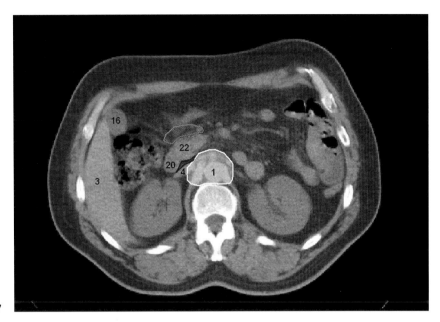

8.27

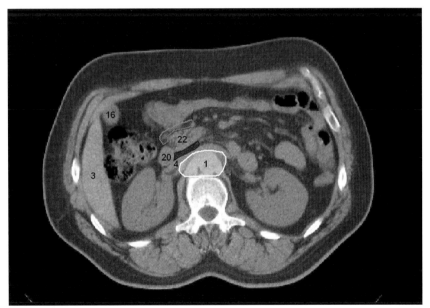

8.28

FIGS. 8.27, 8.28

- POSTERIOR PANCREATICODUODENAL NODES (13)
- NODES AROUND THE ABDOMINAL AORTA (16)
- ANTERIOR PANCREATICODUODENAL NODES (17)

1 – DESCENDING AORTA
3 – LIVER
4 – INFERIOR VENA CAVA
16 – GALLBLADDER
20 – DUODENUM
22 – HEAD OF PANCREAS

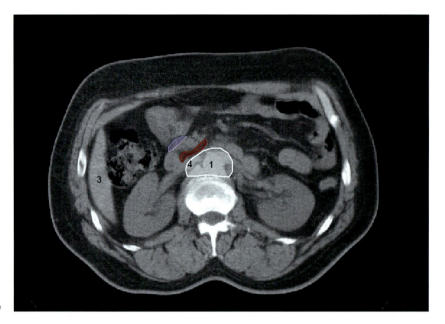

8.29

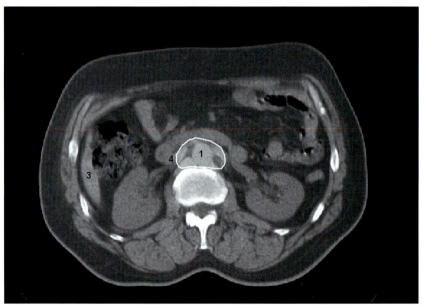

8.30

FIGS. 8.29, 8.30

- POSTERIOR PANCREATICODUODENAL NODES (13)
- NODES AROUND THE ABDOMINAL AORTA (16)
- ANTERIOR PANCREATICODUODENAL NODES (17)

1 – DESCENDING AORTA
3 – LIVER
4 – INFERIOR VENA CAVA

Upper Abdominal Region Lymph Nodes

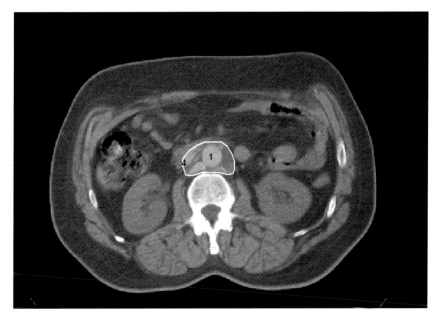

8.31

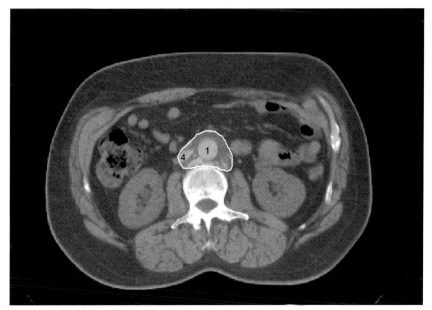

8.32

FIGS. 8.31, 8.32

- NODES AROUND THE ABDOMINAL AORTA (16)

1 – DESCENDING AORTA
4 – INFERIOR VENA CAVA

A Guide for Delineation of Lymph Nodal Clinical Target Volume in Radiation Therapy

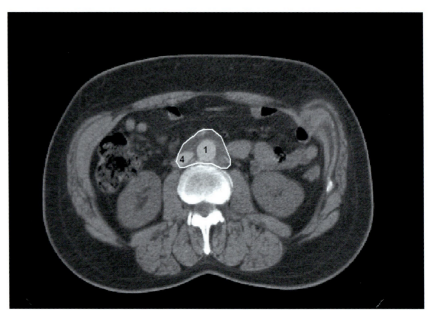

8.33

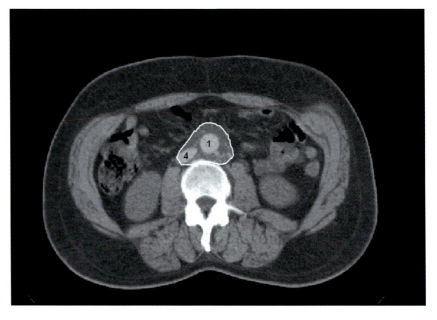

8.34

FIGS. 8.33, 8.34

- NODES AROUND THE ABDOMINAL AORTA (16)

1 – DESCENDING AORTA
4 – INFERIOR VENA CAVA

Upper Abdominal Region Lymph Nodes

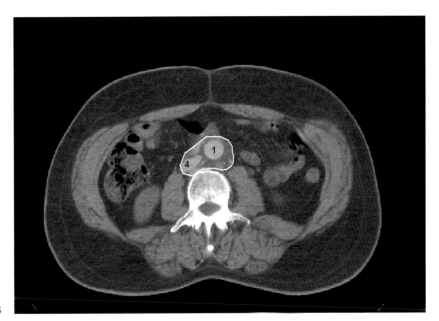

8.35

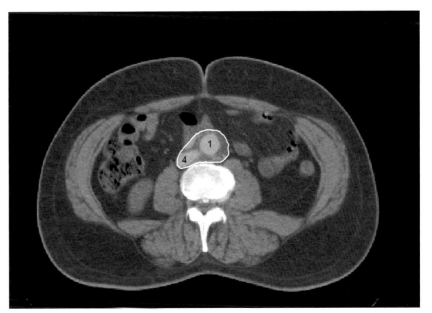

8.36

FIGS. 8.35, 8.36

— NODES AROUND THE ABDOMINAL AORTA (16)

1 – DESCENDING AORTA
4 – INFERIOR VENA CAVA

A Guide for Delineation of Lymph Nodal Clinical Target Volume in Radiation Therapy

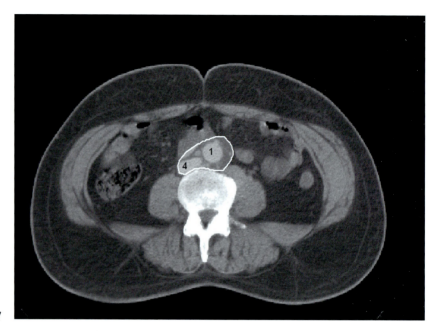

8.37

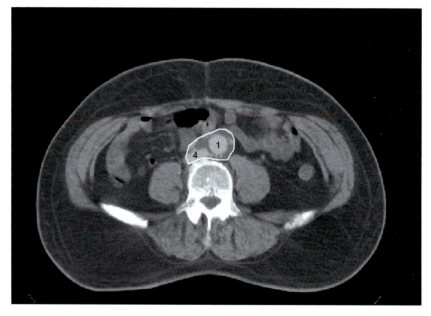

8.38

FIGS. 8.37, 8.38

- NODES AROUND THE ABDOMINAL AORTA (16)

1 – DESCENDING AORTA
4 – INFERIOR VENA CAVA

Upper Abdominal Region Lymph Nodes

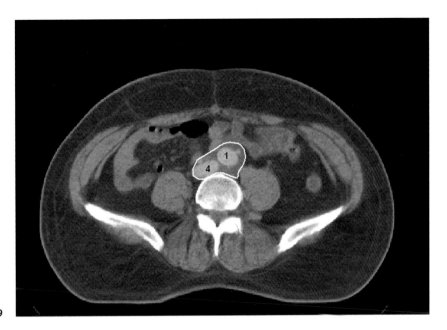

8.39

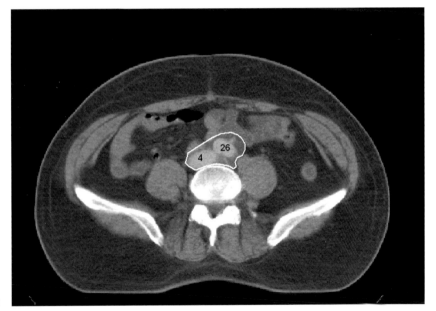

8.40

FIGS. 8.39, 8.40

— NODES AROUND THE ABDOMINAL AORTA (16)

1 – DESCENDING AORTA
4 – INFERIOR VENA CAVA
26 – BIFURCATION OF THE ABDOMINAL AORTA

Pelvic Lymph Nodes

* This chapter has been written with the contributions of Antonietta Augurio, Nicola Filippo Basilico, Antonella Filippone, and Pietro Sanpaolo

A Guide for Delineation of Lymph Nodal Clinical Target Volume in Radiation Therapy

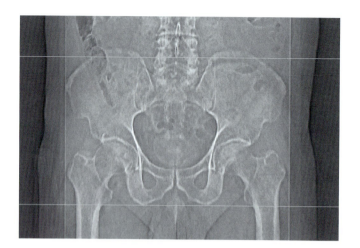

SCOUT VIEW OF PELVIC REGION

Lymph nodes	Anatomical boundaries					
	Cranial	Caudal	Medial	Lateral	Anterior	Posterior
Common iliac nodes	Bifurcation of abdominal aorta (at the inferior border of L4)	Bifurcation of the common iliac vessels (at the inferior border of L5, at the level of the superior border of the ala of sacrum)	Loose cellular tissue	Psoas muscle	Loose cellular tissue anterior to the common iliac vessels	Body of L5
Internal iliac nodes	Bifurcation of common iliac vessels (at the inferior border of L5)	Plane through superior border of the head of femurs at the level of the superior border of the coccyx	Loose cellular tissue	Piriformis muscle	Posterior border of the external iliac lymph nodes and loose cellular tissue	Loose cellular tissue
External iliac nodes	Bifurcation of common iliac vessels (at the inferior border of L5)	Femoral artery	Loose cellular tissue	Iliopsoas muscle	Loose cellular tissue	Anterior border of the internal iliac lymph nodes and loose cellular tissue
Obturator nodes	Plane through the acetabulum	Superior border of the neck of femurs, at the small ischiadic foramen	Loose cellular tissue	Internal obturator muscle (intrapelvic portion)	Loose cellular tissue	Loose cellular tissue
Presacral nodes	Intervertebral space of L5–S1 (sacral promontory)	Superior border of the 1st coccygeal vertebra	–	Piriformis muscle	Loose cellular tissue	Anterior aspect of sacrum
Inguinal nodes	Superior limit of the neck of femurs	Bifurcation of the femoral artery into its superficial and deep branches	Adductor muscles	For superficial inguinal nodes: the adipose and loose connective tissue and the sartorius muscle; for deep inguinal nodes: the femoral vessels	Subcutaneous adipose tissue	Pectineal muscle

A Guide for Delineation of Lymph Nodal Clinical Target Volume in Radiation Therapy

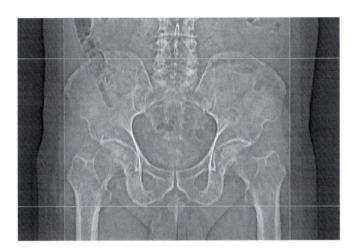

SCOUT VIEW OF PELVIC REGION

Lymph nodes	Anatomical boundaries					
	Cranial	Caudal	Medial	Lateral	Anterior	Posterior
Common iliac nodes	Bifurcation of abdominal aorta (at the inferior border of L4)	Bifurcation of the common iliac vessels (at the inferior border of L5, at the level of the superior border of the ala of sacrum)	Loose cellular tissue	Psoas muscle	Loose cellular tissue anterior to the common iliac vessels	Body of L5
Internal iliac nodes	Bifurcation of common iliac vessels (at the inferior border of L5)	Plane through superior border of the head of femurs at the level of the superior border of the coccyx	Loose cellular tissue	Piriformis muscle	Posterior border of the external iliac lymph nodes and loose cellular tissue	Loose cellular tissue
External iliac nodes	Bifurcation of common iliac vessels (at the inferior border of L5)	Femoral artery	Loose cellular tissue	Iliopsoas muscle	Loose cellular tissue	Anterior border of the internal iliac lymph nodes and loose cellular tissue
Obturator nodes	Plane through the acetabulum	Superior border of the neck of femurs, at the small ischiadic foramen	Loose cellular tissue	Internal obturator muscle (intrapelvic portion)	Loose cellular tissue	Loose cellular tissue
Presacral nodes	Intervertebral space of L5–S1 (sacral promontory)	Superior border of the 1st coccygeal vertebra	–	Piriformis muscle	Loose cellular tissue	Anterior aspect of sacrum
Inguinal nodes	Superior limit of the neck of femurs	Bifurcation of the femoral artery into its superficial and deep branches	Adductor muscles	For superficial inguinal nodes: the adipose and loose connective tissue and the sartorius muscle; for deep inguinal nodes: the femoral vessels	Subcutaneous adipose tissue	Pectineal muscle

Pelvic Lymph Nodes

ANATOMICAL REFERENCE POINTS

1 – RIGHT COMMON ILIAC VEIN
2 – RIGHT COMMON ILIAC ARTERY
3 – LEFT COMMON ILIAC VEIN
4 – LEFT COMMON ILIAC ARTERY
5 – PSOAS MUSCLE
6 – RIGHT COMMON ILIAC ARTERY BIFURCATION
7 – LEFT COMMON ILIAC ARTERY BIFURCATION
8 – CONFLUENCE OF THE RIGHT EXTERNAL AND INTERNAL ILIAC VEINS
9 – LEFT INTERNAL ILIAC ARTERY
10 – LEFT EXTERNAL ILIAC ARTERY
11 – RIGHT EXTERNAL ILIAC VEIN
12 – RIGHT INTERNAL ILIAC VEIN
13 – RIGHT EXTERNAL ILIAC ARTERY
14 – RIGHT INTERNAL ILIAC ARTERY
15 – ILIAC MUSCLE
16 – CONFLUENCE OF THE LEFT EXTERNAL AND INTERNAL ILIAC VEINS
17 – LEFT EXTERNAL ILIAC VEIN
18 – LEFT INTERNAL ILIAC VEIN
19 – ILIOPSOAS MUSCLE
20 – PIRIFORMIS MUSCLE
21 – INTERNAL OBTURATOR MUSCLE
22 – SARTORIUS MUSCLE
23 – RIGHT FEMORAL VEIN
24 – RIGHT FEMORAL ARTERY
25 – LEFT FEMORAL VEIN
26 – LEFT FEMORAL ARTERY
27 – PECTINEAL MUSCLE
28 – RIGHT DEEP FEMORAL ARTERY
29 – LEFT DEEP FEMORAL ARTERY
30 – GREAT SAPHENOUS VEIN
31 – ANAL VERGE

COLOR LEGEND

- COMMON ILIAC NODES
- INTERNAL ILIAC NODES
- EXTERNAL ILIAC NODES
- PRESACRAL NODES
- OBTURATOR NODES
- INGUINAL NODES

A Guide for Delineation of Lymph Nodal Clinical Target Volume in Radiation Therapy

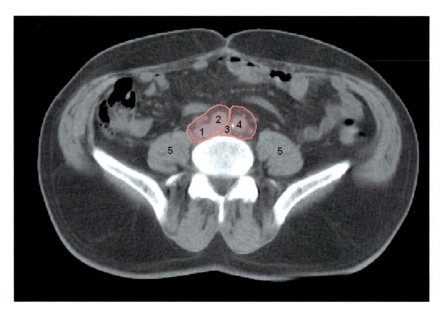

9.1

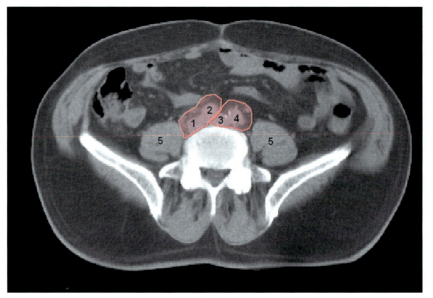

9.2

FIGS. 9.1, 9.2

■ COMMON ILIAC NODES

1 – RIGHT COMMON ILIAC VEIN
2 – RIGHT COMMON ILIAC ARTERY
3 – LEFT COMMON ILIAC VEIN
4 – LEFT COMMON ILIAC ARTERY
5 – PSOAS MUSCLE

Pelvic Lymph Nodes

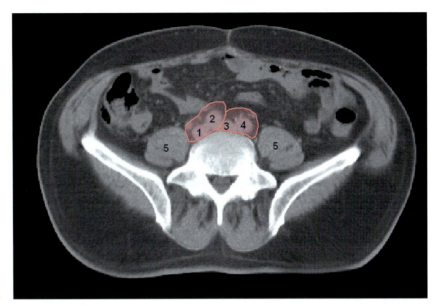

9.3

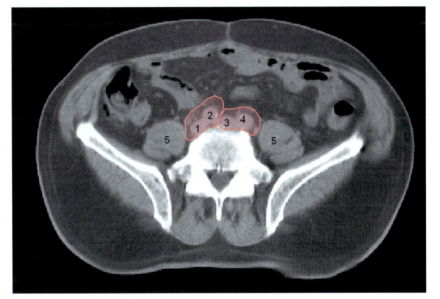

9.4

FIGS. 9.3, 9.4

— COMMON ILIAC NODES

1 – RIGHT COMMON ILIAC VEIN
2 – RIGHT COMMON ILIAC ARTERY
3 – LEFT COMMON ILIAC VEIN
4 – LEFT COMMON ILIAC ARTERY
5 – PSOAS MUSCLE

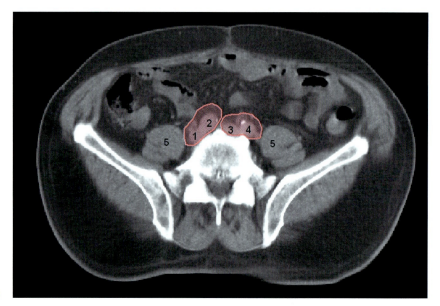

9.5

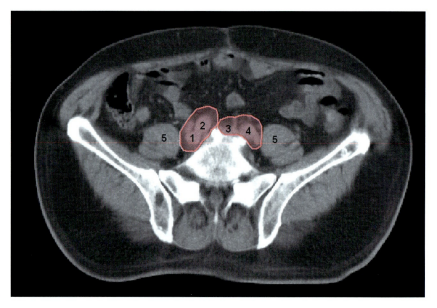

9.6

FIGS. 9.5, 9.6

■ COMMON ILIAC NODES

1 – RIGHT COMMON ILIAC VEIN
2 – RIGHT COMMON ILIAC ARTERY
3 – LEFT COMMON ILIAC VEIN
4 – LEFT COMMON ILIAC ARTERY
5 – PSOAS MUSCLE

Pelvic Lymph Nodes

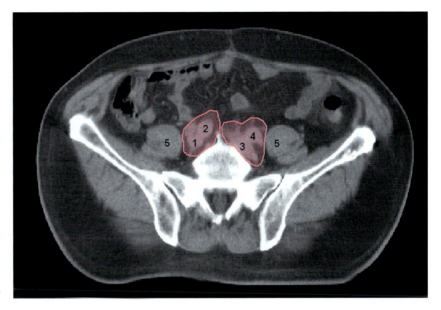

9.7

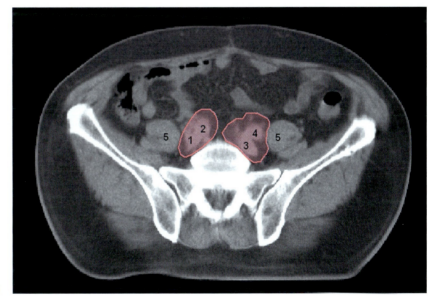

9.8

FIGS. 9.7, 9.8

— COMMON ILIAC NODES

1 – RIGHT COMMON ILIAC VEIN
2 – RIGHT COMMON ILIAC ARTERY
3 – LEFT COMMON ILIAC VEIN
4 – LEFT COMMON ILIAC ARTERY
5 – PSOAS MUSCLE

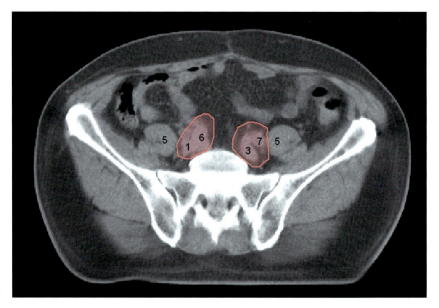

9.9

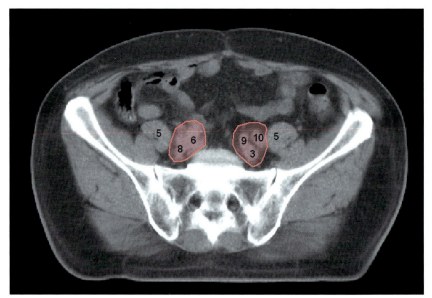

9.10

FIGS. 9.9, 9.10

— COMMON ILIAC NODES

1 – RIGHT COMMON ILIAC VEIN
3 – LEFT COMMON ILIAC VEIN
5 – PSOAS MUSCLE
6 – RIGHT COMMON ILIAC ARTERY BIFURCATION
7 – LEFT COMMON ILIAC ARTERY BIFURCATION
8 – CONFLUENCE OF THE RIGHT EXTERNAL AND INTERNAL ILIAC VEINS
9 – LEFT INTERNAL ILIAC ARTERY
10 – LEFT EXTERNAL ILIAC ARTERY

Pelvic Lymph Nodes

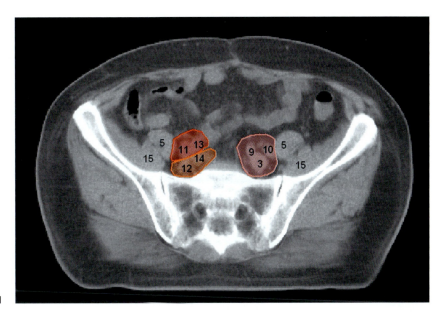

9.11

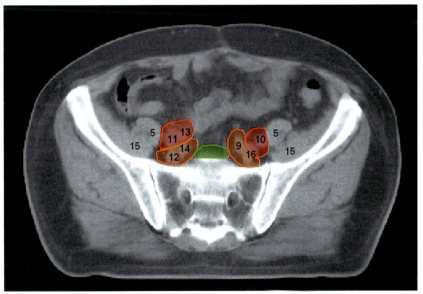

9.12

FIGS. 9.11, 9.12
- COMMON ILIAC NODES
- INTERNAL ILIAC NODES
- EXTERNAL ILIAC NODES
- PRESACRAL NODES

3 – LEFT COMMON ILIAC VEIN
5 – PSOAS MUSCLE
9 – LEFT INTERNAL ILIAC ARTERY
10 – LEFT EXTERNAL ILIAC ARTERY
11 – RIGHT EXTERNAL ILIAC VEIN
12 – RIGHT INTERNAL ILIAC VEIN
13 – RIGHT EXTERNAL ILIAC ARTERY
14 – RIGHT INTERNAL ILIAC ARTERY
15 – ILIAC MUSCLE
16 – CONFLUENCE OF THE LEFT EXTERNAL AND INTERNAL ILIAC VEINS

A Guide for Delineation of Lymph Nodal Clinical Target Volume in Radiation Therapy

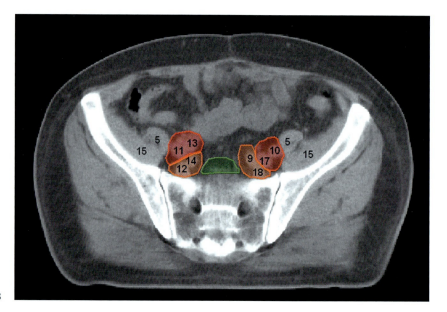

9.13

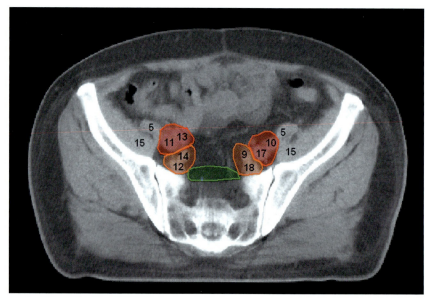

9.14

FIGS. 9.13, 9.14
- INTERNAL ILIAC NODES
- EXTERNAL ILIAC NODES
- PRESACRAL NODES

5 – PSOAS MUSCLE
9 – LEFT INTERNAL ILIAC ARTERY
10 – LEFT EXTERNAL ILIAC ARTERY
11 – RIGHT EXTERNAL ILIAC VEIN
12 – RIGHT INTERNAL ILIAC VEIN
13 – RIGHT EXTERNAL ILIAC ARTERY
14 – RIGHT INTERNAL ILIAC ARTERY
15 – ILIAC MUSCLE
17 – LEFT EXTERNAL ILIAC VEIN
18 – LEFT INTERNAL ILIAC VEIN

Pelvic Lymph Nodes

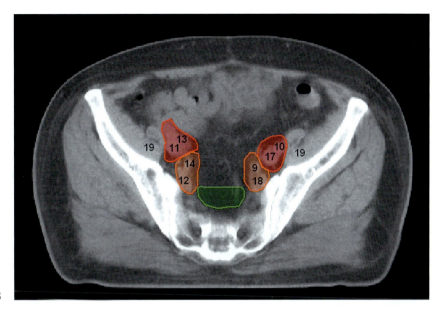

9.15

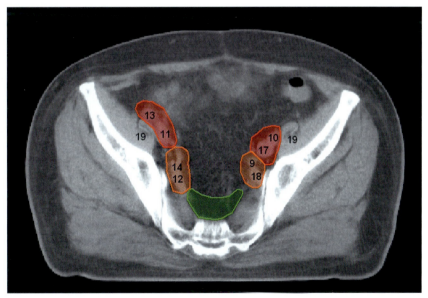

9.16

FIGS. 9.15, 9.16
- INTERNAL ILIAC NODES
- EXTERNAL ILIAC NODES
- PRESACRAL NODES

9 – LEFT INTERNAL ILIAC ARTERY
10 – LEFT EXTERNAL ILIAC ARTERY
11 – RIGHT EXTERNAL ILIAC VEIN
12 – RIGHT INTERNAL ILIAC VEIN
13 – RIGHT EXTERNAL ILIAC ARTERY
14 – RIGHT INTERNAL ILIAC ARTERY
17 – LEFT EXTERNAL ILIAC VEIN
18 – LEFT INTERNAL ILIAC VEIN
19 – ILIOPSOAS MUSCLE

A Guide for Delineation of Lymph Nodal Clinical Target Volume in Radiation Therapy

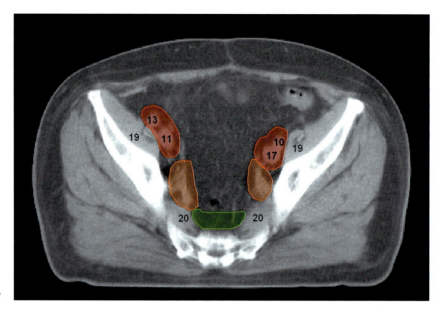

9.17

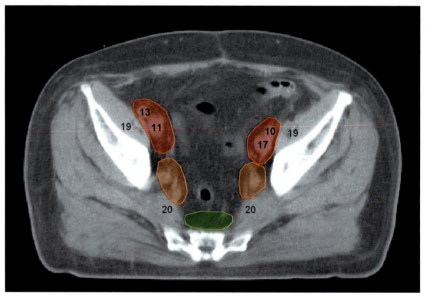

9.18

FIGS. 9.17, 9.18

- INTERNAL ILIAC NODES
- EXTERNAL ILIAC NODES
- PRESACRAL NODES

10 – LEFT EXTERNAL ILIAC ARTERY
11 – RIGHT EXTERNAL ILIAC VEIN
13 – RIGHT EXTERNAL ILIAC ARTERY
17 – LEFT EXTERNAL ILIAC VEIN
19 – ILIOPSOAS MUSCLE
20 – PIRIFORMIS MUSCLE

Pelvic Lymph Nodes

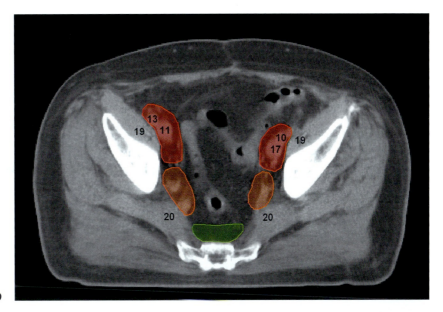

9.19

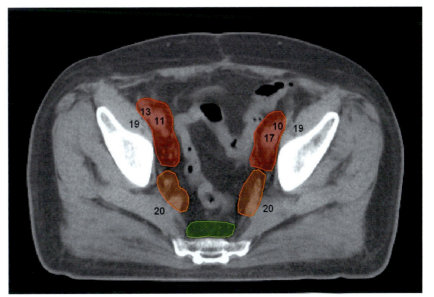

9.20

FIGS. 9.19, 9.20
- INTERNAL ILIAC NODES
- EXTERNAL ILIAC NODES
- PRESACRAL NODES

10 – LEFT EXTERNAL ILIAC ARTERY
11 – RIGHT EXTERNAL ILIAC VEIN
13 – RIGHT EXTERNAL ILIAC ARTERY
17 – LEFT EXTERNAL ILIAC VEIN
19 – ILIOPSOAS MUSCLE
20 – PIRIFORMIS MUSCLE

A Guide for Delineation of Lymph Nodal Clinical Target Volume in Radiation Therapy

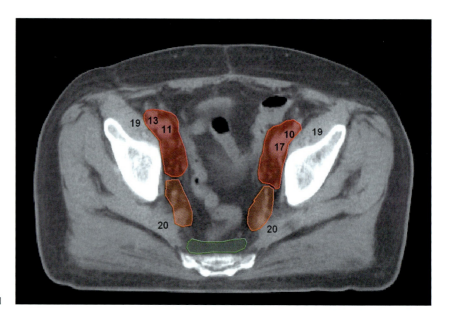

9.21

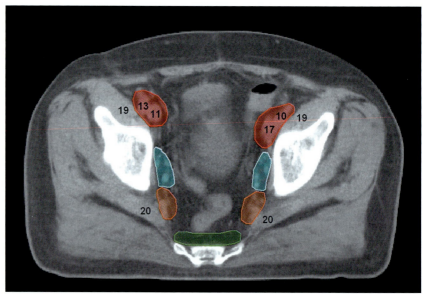

9.22

FIGS. 9.21, 9.22

- INTERNAL ILIAC NODES
- EXTERNAL ILIAC NODES
- PRESACRAL NODES
- OBTURATOR NODES

10 – LEFT EXTERNAL ILIAC ARTERY
11 – RIGHT EXTERNAL ILIAC VEIN
13 – RIGHT EXTERNAL ILIAC ARTERY
17 – LEFT EXTERNAL ILIAC VEIN
19 – ILIOPSOAS MUSCLE
20 – PIRIFORMIS MUSCLE

Pelvic Lymph Nodes

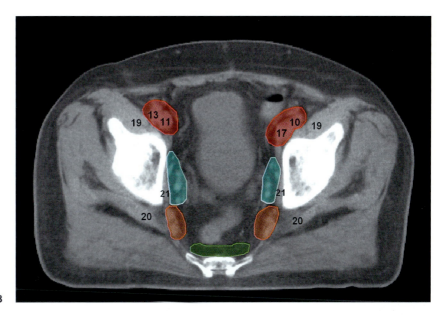

9.23

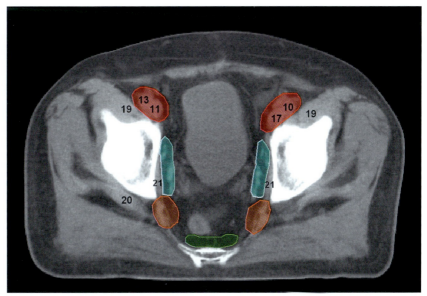

9.24

FIGS. 9.23, 9.24
- INTERNAL ILIAC NODES
- EXTERNAL ILIAC NODES
- PRESACRAL NODES
- OBTURATOR NODES

10 – LEFT EXTERNAL ILIAC ARTERY
11 – RIGHT EXTERNAL ILIAC VEIN
13 – RIGHT EXTERNAL ILIAC ARTERY
17 – LEFT EXTERNAL ILIAC VEIN
19 – ILIOPSOAS MUSCLE
20 – PIRIFORMIS MUSCLE
21 – INTERNAL OBTURATOR MUSCLE

A Guide for Delineation of Lymph Nodal Clinical Target Volume in Radiation Therapy

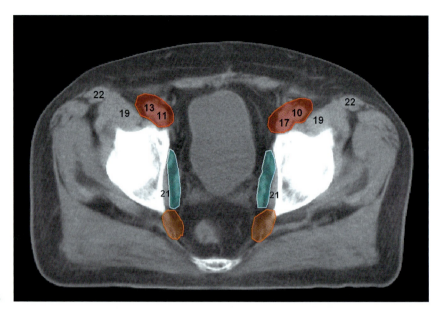

9.25

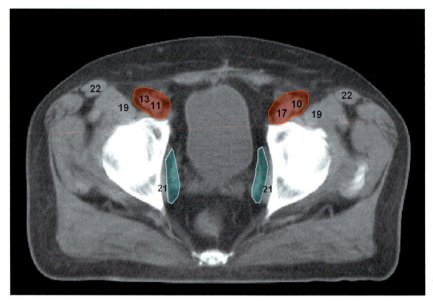

9.26

FIGS. 9.25, 9.26

- INTERNAL ILIAC NODES
- EXTERNAL ILIAC NODES
- OBTURATOR NODES

10 – LEFT EXTERNAL ILIAC ARTERY
11 – RIGHT EXTERNAL ILIAC VEIN
13 – RIGHT EXTERNAL ILIAC ARTERY
17 – LEFT EXTERNAL ILIAC VEIN
19 – ILIOPSOAS MUSCLE
21 – INTERNAL OBTURATOR MUSCLE
22 – SARTORIUS MUSCLE

Pelvic Lymph Nodes

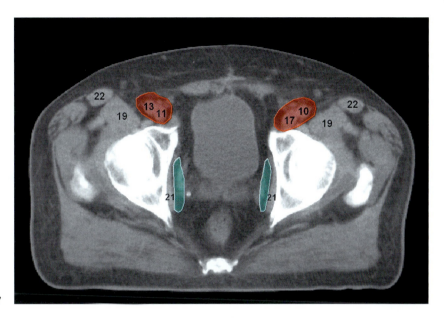

9.27

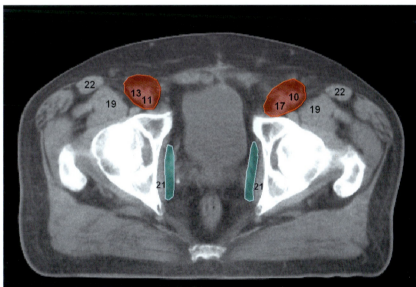

9.28

FIGS. 9.27, 9.28
- EXTERNAL ILIAC NODES
- OBTURATOR NODES

10 – LEFT EXTERNAL ILIAC ARTERY
11 – RIGHT EXTERNAL ILIAC VEIN
13 – RIGHT EXTERNAL ILIAC ARTERY
17 – LEFT EXTERNAL ILIAC VEIN
19 – ILIOPSOAS MUSCLE
21 – INTERNAL OBTURATOR MUSCLE
22 – SARTORIUS MUSCLE

A Guide for Delineation of Lymph Nodal Clinical Target Volume in Radiation Therapy

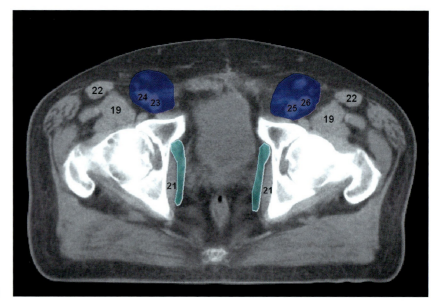

9.29

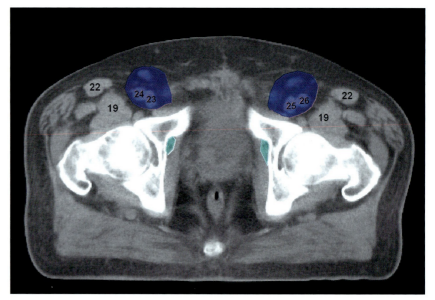

9.30

FIGS. 9.29, 9.30

- OBTURATOR NODES
- INGUINAL NODES

19 – ILIOPSOAS MUSCLE
21 – INTERNAL OBTURATOR MUSCLE
22 – SARTORIUS MUSCLE
23 – RIGHT FEMORAL VEIN
24 – RIGHT FEMORAL ARTERY
25 – LEFT FEMORAL VEIN
26 – LEFT FEMORAL ARTERY

Pelvic Lymph Nodes

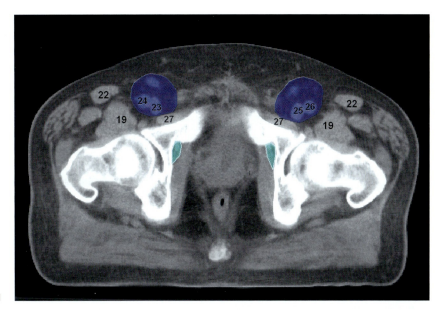

9.31

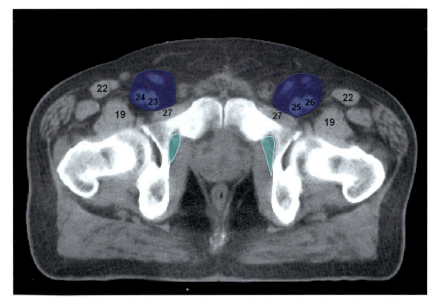

9.32

FIGS. 9.31, 9.32
- OBTURATOR NODES
- INGUINAL NODES

19 – ILIOPSOAS MUSCLE
22 – SARTORIUS MUSCLE
23 – RIGHT FEMORAL VEIN
24 – RIGHT FEMORAL ARTERY
25 – LEFT FEMORAL VEIN
26 – LEFT FEMORAL ARTERY
27 – PECTINEAL MUSCLE

A Guide for Delineation of Lymph Nodal Clinical Target Volume in Radiation Therapy

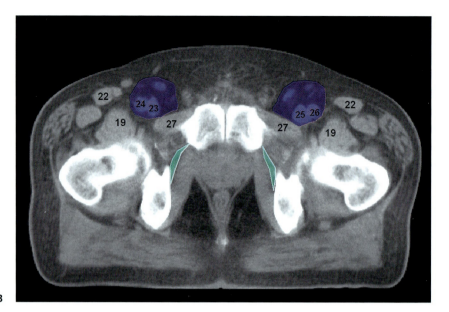

9.33

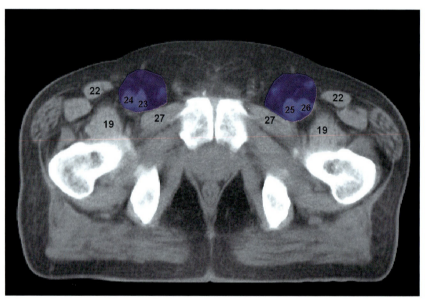

9.34

FIGS. 9.33, 9.34

- OBTURATOR NODES
- INGUINAL NODES

19 – ILIOPSOAS MUSCLE
22 – SARTORIUS MUSCLE
23 – RIGHT FEMORAL VEIN
24 – RIGHT FEMORAL ARTERY
25 – LEFT FEMORAL VEIN
26 – LEFT FEMORAL ARTERY
27 – PECTINEAL MUSCLE

Pelvic Lymph Nodes

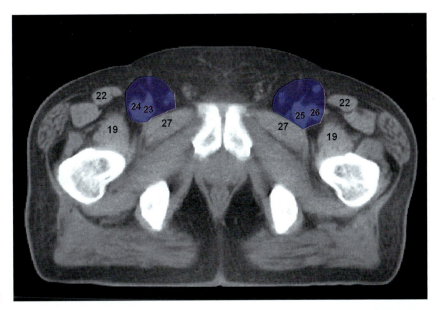

9.35

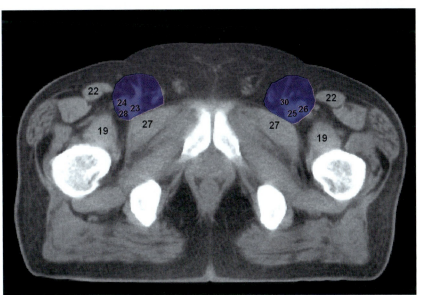

9.36

FIGS. 9.35, 9.36
— INGUINAL NODES

19 – ILIOPSOAS MUSCLE
22 – SARTORIUS MUSCLE
23 – RIGHT FEMORAL VEIN
24 – RIGHT FEMORAL ARTERY
25 – LEFT FEMORAL VEIN
26 – LEFT FEMORAL ARTERY
27 – PECTINEAL MUSCLE
28 – RIGHT DEEP FEMORAL ARTERY
30 – GREAT SAPHENOUS VEIN

A Guide for Delineation of Lymph Nodal Clinical Target Volume in Radiation Therapy

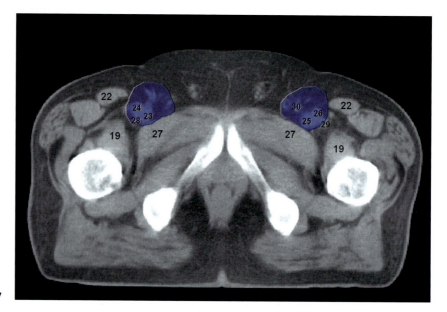

9.37

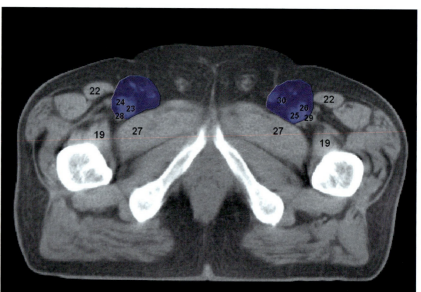

9.38

FIGS. 9.37, 9.38

▬ INGUINAL NODES

19 – ILIOPSOAS MUSCLE
22 – SARTORIUS MUSCLE
23 – RIGHT FEMORAL VEIN
24 – RIGHT FEMORAL ARTERY
25 – LEFT FEMORAL VEIN
26 – LEFT FEMORAL ARTERY
27 – PECTINEAL MUSCLE
28 – RIGHT DEEP FEMORAL ARTERY
29 – LEFT DEEP FEMORAL ARTERY
30 – GREAT SAPHENOUS VEIN

Pelvic Lymph Nodes

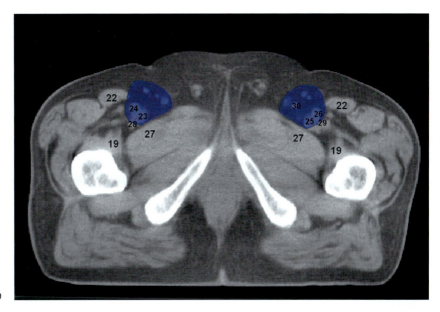

9.39

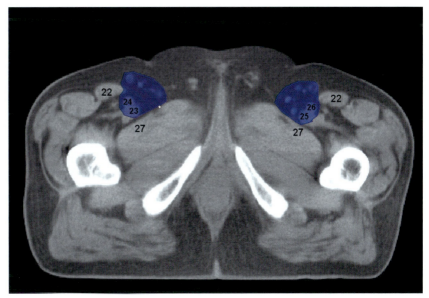

9.40

FIGS. 9.39, 9.40
▬ INGUINAL NODES

19 – ILIOPSOAS MUSCLE
22 – SARTORIUS MUSCLE
23 – RIGHT FEMORAL VEIN
24 – RIGHT FEMORAL ARTERY
25 – LEFT FEMORAL VEIN
26 – LEFT FEMORAL ARTERY
27 – PECTINEAL MUSCLE
28 – RIGHT DEEP FEMORAL ARTERY
29 – LEFT DEEP FEMORAL ARTERY
30 – GREAT SAPHENOUS VEIN

A Guide for Delineation of Lymph Nodal Clinical Target Volume in Radiation Therapy

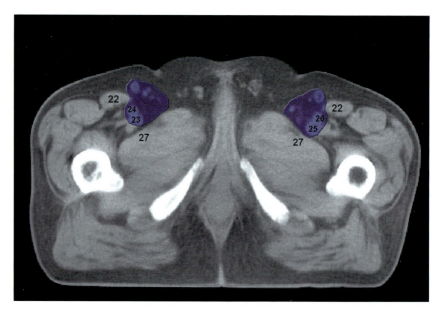

9.41

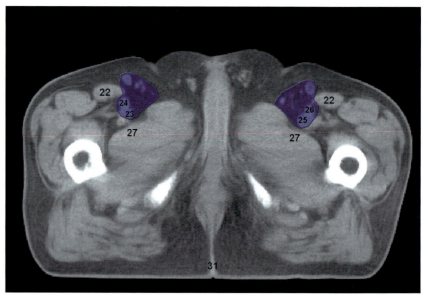

9.42

FIGS. 9.41, 9.42

▬ INGUINAL NODES

22 – SARTORIUS MUSCLE
23 – RIGHT FEMORAL VEIN
24 – RIGHT FEMORAL ARTERY
25 – LEFT FEMORAL VEIN
26 – LEFT FEMORAL ARTERY
27 – PECTINEAL MUSCLE
31 – ANAL VERGE

Digitally Reconstructed Radiographs (DRRs)

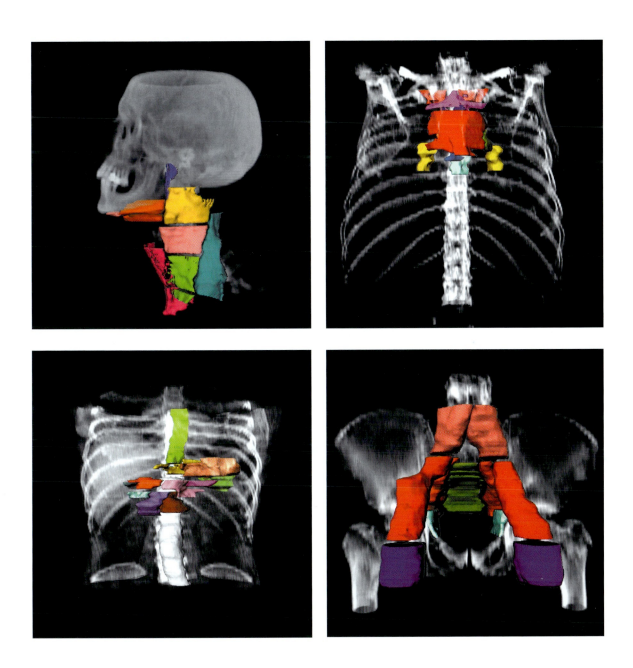

References

1. Testut L, Latarjet A (1972) Trattato di anatomia umana, 5th edn. UTET, Torino
2. Rouvière H (1938) Lymphatic system of the head and neck. Tobias MJ (translator). Edwards, Ann Arbor
3. Rouvière H (1967) Anatomie humaine, descriptive et topographique. Masson, Paris
4. Park JM, Charnsangavej C, Yoshimitsu K, Herron DH, Robinson TJ, Wallace S (1994) Pathways of nodal metastasis from pelvic tumours: CT demonstration. Radiographics 14:1309–1321
5. Pannu HK, Corl FM, Fishman EK (2001) CT evaluation of cervical cancer: spectrum of disease. Radiographics 21:1155–1168
6. Gregoire V, Scalliet P, Ang KK (eds) (2004) Clinical target volumes in conformal and intensity modulated radiation therapy. A clinical guide to cancer treatment. Springer, Berlin
7. International Commission of Radiation Units and Measurements (1993) Prescribing, recording and reporting photon beam therapy. ICRU report 50. ICRU, Bethesda
8. International Commission of Radiation Units and Measurements (1999) Prescribing, recording and reporting photon beam therapy (supplement to ICRU report 50). ICRU report 62, ICRU, Bethesda
9. Trotter H (1930) The surgical anatomy of the lymphatics of the head and neck. Ann Otol Rhinol Laryngol 39:384–397
10. Poirer P, Charpy A (1909) Traité d'anatomie humaine, vol 2, 2nd edn. Paris
11. Mancuso AA, Harnsberger HR, Muraki AS, Stevens MH (1983) Computed tomography of cervical and retropharyngeal lymph nodes: normal anatomy, variants of normal, and application in staging head and neck cancer, part II: pathology. Radiology 148:715–723
12. Spiro RH (1985) The management of neck nodes in head and neck cancer: a surgeon's view. Bull N Y Acad Med 61:629–637
13. Medina JE (1989) A rational classification of neck dissections. Otolaryngol Head Neck Surg 100:169–176
14. Beahrs OH, Henson DE, Hutter RVP, Meyers MH (eds) (1988) American Joint Committee on Cancer. Manual for staging cancer, 3rd edn. Lippincott, Philadelphia
15. Shah JP, Strong E, Spiro RH, Vikram B (1981) Surgical grand rounds. Neck dissection: current status and future possibilities. Clin Bull 11:25–33
16. Robbins KT, Medina JE, Wolfe GT, Levine PA, Sessions RB, Pruet CW (1991) Standardizing neck dissection terminology. Official report of the Academy's Committee for Head and Neck Surgery and Oncology. Arch Otolaryngol Head Neck Surg 117:601–605
17. Hermanek P, Henson DE, Hutter RVP, Sobin LH (eds) (1993) International Union Against

Cancer (UICC): TNM supplement 1993. A commentary on uniform use. Springer, Berlin, pp 19–228
18. Spiessl B, Beahrs OH, Hermanek P et al (1992) TNM atlas. Illustrated guide to the TNM/pTNM classification of malignant tumours, 3rd edn, 2nd revision. Springer, Berlin, pp 4–5
19. American Joint Committee on Cancer (1997) AJCC cancer staging manual, 5th edn. Lippincott-Raven, Philadelphia
20. Robbins KT (1998) Classification of neck dissection: current concepts and future considerations. Otolaryngol Clin North Am 31:639–655
21. Robbins KT (1999) Integrating radiological criteria into the classification of cervical lymph node disease. Arch Otolaryngol Head Neck Surg 125:385–387
22. Robbins KT, Clayman G, Levine PA et al (2002) Neck dissection classification update: revisions proposed by the American Head and Neck Society and the American Academy of Otolaryngology-Head and Neck Surgery. Arch Otolaryngol Head Neck Surg 128:751–758
23. Robbins KT, Atkinson JLD, Byers RM, Cohen JI, Lavertu P, Pellitteri P (2001) The use and misuse of neck dissection for head and neck cancer. J Am Coll Surg 193:91–102
24. Hamoir M, Desuter G, Gregoire V, Reychler H, Rombaux P, Lengele B (2002) A proposal for redefining the boundaries of level V in the neck: is dissection of the apex of level V necessary in mucosal squamous cell carcinoma of the head and neck? Arch Otolaryngol Head Neck Surg 128:1381–1383
25. Suen JY, Goepfert H (1987) Standardization of neck dissection nomenclature. Head Neck Surg 10:75–77
26. Gregoire V, Coche E, Cosnard G, Hamoir M, Reychler H (2000) Selection and delineation of lymph node target volumes in head and neck conformal radiotherapy. Proposal for standardizing terminology and procedure based on the surgical experience. Radiother Oncol 56:135–150
27. Byers RM, Weber RS, Andrews T, McGill D, Kare R, Wolf P (1997) Frequency and therapeutic implications of "skip metastases" in the neck from squamous carcinoma of the oral tongue. Head Neck 19:14–19
28. Naruke T, Suemasu K, Ishikawa S (1976) Surgical treatment for lung cancer with metastasis to mediastinal lymph nodes. J Thorac Cardiovasc Surg 71:279–285
29. Naruke T, Suemasu K, Ishikawa S (1978) Lymph node mapping and curability of various levels of metastases in resected lung cancer. J Thorac Cardiovasc Surg 76:832–839
30. Naruke T (1993) Significance of lymph node metastases in lung cancer. Semin Thorac Cardiovasc Surg 5:210–218
31. Beahrs OH, Hensen DE, Hutter RV, Kennedy BJ (eds) (1992) American Joint Committee on Cancer (AJCC). Lung. Manual for staging of cancer, vol 4. Lippincott, Philadelphia, pp 115–122
32. American Thoracic Society (1983) Medical section of the American Lung Association. Clinical staging of primary lung cancer. Am Rev Respir Dis 127:659–664
33. Glazer GM, Gross BH, Quint LE, Francis IR, Bookstein FL, Orringer MB. Normal mediastinal lymph nodes: number and size according to American Thoracic Society mapping. AJR Am J Roentgenol 144:261–265
34. McLoud TC, Bourguin PM, Greenberg RW et al (1992) Bronchogenic carcinoma: analysis of staging in the mediastinum with CT by correlative lymph node mapping and sampling. Radiology 182:319–323
35. Scott WJ, Gobar LS, Terry JD, Dewan NA, Sunderland JJ (1996) Mediastinal lymph node staging of non-small cell lung cancer: a prospective comparison of computed tomography and positron emission tomography. J Thorac Cardiovasc Surg 111:642–648

References

36. Murray JG, Breatnach E (1993) The American Thoracic Society lymph node map: a CT demonstration. Eur J Radiol 17:61–68
37. The Japan Lung Cancer Society (2000) Classification of lung cancer, 1st English edn. Kanehara, Tokyo
38. American Joint Committee on Cancer (1979) Task force on lung staging of lung cancer 1979. American Joint Committee on Cancer, Chicago, p 23
39. Mountain CF (1997) Revision in the international system for staging lung cancer. Chest 111:1710–1717
40. Mountain CF, Dresler CM (1997) Regional lymph node classification for lung cancer staging. Chest 111:1718–1723
41. Japanese Society for Esophageal Disease (1976) Guidelines for the clinical and pathologic studies for carcinoma of the esophagus, part I: clinical classification. Surg Today 6:79–86
42. Bumm R, Wong J (1994) More or less surgery for esophageal cancer: extent of lymphadenectomy in esophagectomy for squamous cell esophageal carcinoma: how much is necessary? Dis Esophag 7:151–155
43. Mardiros Herbella FA, Del Grande JC, Colleoni R (2003) Anatomical analysis of the mediastinal lymph nodes of normal Brazilian subjects according to the classification of the Japanese Society for Disease of the Esophagus. Surg Today 33:249–253
44. Akiyama H (1990) Surgery for cancer of the esophagus. Williams and Wilkins, Baltimore
45. Casson AG (1994) Lymph node mapping of esophageal cancer. Ann Thorac Surg 58:1569–1570
46. Japanese Research Society for Gastric Cancer (1995) Japanese classification of gastric carcinoma, 1st English edn. Kanehara, Tokyo
47. Japanese Research Society for Gastric Cancer (1993) The general rules for gastric cancer study, 12th edn (in Japanese). Kanehara, Tokyo
48. Japanese Gastric Cancer Association (1998) Japanese classification of gastric carcinoma, 13th edn (in Japanese). Kanehara, Tokyo
49. Japanese Gastric Cancer Association (1998) Japanese classification of gastric carcinoma, 2nd English edn. Gastric Cancer 1:10–24
50. Aiko T, Sasako M, for the General Rules Committee of the Japanese Gastric Cancer Association (1998) The new Japanese classification of gastric carcinoma: points to be revised. Gastric Cancer 1:25–30
51. Japan Pancreas Society (1980) General rules for surgical and pathological studies on cancer of pancreas (in Japanese). Kanehara, Tokyo
52. Liver Cancer Study Group of Japan (1989) The general rules for the clinical and pathological study of primary liver cancer. Jap J Surg 19:98–129
53. Japan Pancreas Society (1982) General rules for surgical and pathological studies on cancer of pancreas, 2nd edn (in Japanese). Kanehara, Tokyo
54. Japan Pancreas Society (1986) General rules for surgical and pathological studies on cancer of pancreas, 3rd edn (in Japanese). Kanehara, Tokyo
55. Japan Pancreas Society (1993) General rules for surgical and pathological studies on cancer of pancreas, 4th edn (in Japanese). Kanehara, Tokyo
56. Japan Pancreas Society (1996) Classification of pancreatic carcinoma, 1st English edn. Kanehara, Tokyo
57. Sobin LH, Wittekind C (eds) (1997) TNM classification of malignant tumours: International Union Against Cancer, 5th edn. Wiley, New York
58. Kawarada Y (2003) New classification of pancreatic carcinoma. Japan Pancreas Society Nippon Shokakibyo Gakkai Zasshi 100:974–980
59. Kawarada Y (2006) JPS, 5th edn. Classification of pancreatic cancer and JPS classification

versus UICC classification. Nippon Rinsho 64 (suppl 1):81–86
60. Kawarada Y, Yamagiwa K, Isaji S, Mizu-moto R (1994) The prevalence of pancreatic cancer lymph node metastasis in Japan and pancreatic staging categories. Int J Pancreatol 16:101–104
61. Pedrazzoli S, Beger HG, Obertop H et al (1999) A surgical and pathological based classification of resective treatment of pancreatic cancer. Summary of an international workshop on surgical procedures in pancreatic cancer. Dig Surg 16:337–345
62. Reiffenstuhl G (1964) The lymphatics of the female genital organs. Lippincott, Philadelphia
63. Plentl AA, Friedman EA (1971) Lymphatic system of the female genitalia. Saunders, Philadelphia
64. Mangan C, Rubin S, Rabin D, Mikuta JJ (1986) Lymph node nomenclature in gynecologic oncology. Gynecol Oncol 23:222–226
65. Benedetti Panici PL, Scambia G, Baiocchi G (1992) Anatomical study of para-aortic and pelvic lymph nodes in gynecologic malignancies. Obstet Gynecol 79:498–502
66. Valentini V, Dinapoli N, Nori S et al (2004) An application of visible human database in radiotherapy: tutorial for image guided external radiotherapy (TIGER). Radiother Oncol 70:165–169
67. Nowak PJCM, Wijers OB, Lagerwaard FJ, Levendag PC (1999) A three-dimensional CT-based target definition for elective irradiation of the neck. Int J Radiat Oncol Biol Phys 45:33–39
68. Som PM, Curtin HD, Mancuso AA (1999) An imaging-based classification for the cervical nodes designed as an adjunct to recent clinically based nodal classifications. Arch Otolaryngol Head Neck Surg 125:388–396
69. Som PM, Curtin HD, Mancuso AA (2000) Imaging-based nodal classification for evaluation of neck metastatic adenopathy. AJR Am J Roentgenol 174:837–844
70. Hayman LA, Taber KH, Diaz-Marchan PJ, Stewart MG, Malcolm ML, Laine FJ (1998) Spatial compartments of the neck, part III: axial sections. Int J Neuroradiol 4:393–402
71. Stewart MG, Hayman LA, Taber KH, Diaz-Marchan PJ, Laine FJ (1998) Clinical pathology of the neck: spatial compartments. Int J Neuroradiol 4:152–158
72. Martinez-Monge R, Fernandes PS, Gupta N, Gahbauer R (1999) Cross-sectional nodal atlas: a tool for the definition of clinical target volumes in three-dimensional radiation therapy planning. Radiology 211:815–828
73. Wijers OB, Levendag PC, Tan T et al (1999) A simplified CT-based definition of the lymph node levels in the node negative neck. Radiother Oncol 52:35–42
74. Chao KS, Wippold FJ, Ozyigit G, Tran BN, Dempsey JF (2002) Determination and delineation of nodal target volumes for head-and-neck cancer based on patterns of failure in patients receiving definitive and postoperative IMRT. Int J Radiat Oncol Biol Phys 53:1174–1184
75. Palazzi M, Barsacchi L, Bianchi E et al (2000) Three-dimensional CT-based contouring of nodal levels in the neck: results of a multicenter dummy-run study by the AIRO – Lombardia Cooperative Group. Radiother Oncol 56(S1):A592
76. Palazzi M, Soatti C, Bianchi E et al, on behalf of the AIRO – Lombardia Head and Neck Working Party (2002) Guidelines for the delineation of nodal regions of the head and neck on axial computed tomography images. Tumori 88:355–360
77. Levendag P, Braaksma M, Coche E et al (2004) Rotterdam and Brussels CT-based neck nodal delineation compared with the surgical levels as defined by the American Academy of Otolaryngology-Head and Neck Surgery. Int J Radiat Oncol Biol Phys 58:113–123

78. Gregoire V, Levendag P, Ang KK et al (2003) CT-based delineation of lymph node levels and related CTVs in the node-negative neck: DAHANCA, EORTC, GOERTEC, NCIC, RTOG consensus guidelines. Radiother Oncol 69:227–236
79. Levendag P, Gregoire V, Hamoir M et al (2005) Intraoperative validation of CT-based lymph nodal levels, sublevels IIA and IIB: is it of clinical relevance in selective radiation therapy? Int J Radiat Oncol Biol Phys 62:690–699
80. Senan S, De Ruysscher D, Giraud P, Mirimanoff R, Budach V, on behalf of the Radiotherapy Group of the European Organization for Research and Treatment of Cancer (EORTC) (2004) Literature-based recommendations for treatment planning and execution in high-dose radiotherapy for lung cancer. Radiother Oncol 7:139–146
81. Cymbalista M, Waysberg A, Zacharias C et al (1999) CT demonstration of the 1996 AJCC-UICC regional lymph node classification for lung cancer staging. Radiographics 19:899–900
82. Vinciguerra A, Taraborrelli M, D'Alessandro M, Barbieri V, Ausili Cefaro G (2003) Contouring of lymph nodal clinical target volume (CTVs) in lung cancer radiation therapy: Chieti experience. Tumori 2:S76
83. Chapet O, Kong FM, Quint LE et al (2005) CT-based definition of thoracic lymph node stations: an atlas from the University of Michigan. Int J Radiat Oncol Biol Phys 63:170–178
84. Cellini F, Valentini V, Pacelli F et al (2003) Preoperative radiotherapy in gastric cancer: CTV definition for conformal therapy according to tumor location. Rays 28:317–329
85. Greer BE, Koh W-J, Figge DC, Russell AH, Cain JM, Tamimi HK (1990) Gynecologic radiotherapy fields defined by intraoperative measurements. Gynecol Oncol 38:421–424
86. Bonin SR, Lanciano RM, Corn BW, Hogan WM, Hartz WH, Hanks GE (1996) Bony landmarks are not an adequate substitute for lymphangiography in defining pelvic lymph node location for the treatment of cervical cancer with radiotherapy. Int J Radiat Oncol Biol Phys 34:167–172
87. Zunino S, Rosato O, Lucino S, Jauregui E, Rossi L, Venencia D (1999) Anatomic study of the pelvis in carcinoma of the uterine cervix as related to the box technique. Int J Radiat Oncol Biol Phys 44:53–59
88. Roeske JC, Lujan A, Rotmensch J, Waggoner SE, Yamada D, Mundt AJ (2000) Intensity-modulated whole pelvic radiation therapy in patients with gynecologic malignancies. Int J Radiat Oncol Biol Phys 48:1613–1621
89. Nutting CM, Convery DJ, Cosgrove VP et al (2000) Reduction of small and large bowel irradiation using an optimized intensity-modulated pelvic radiotherapy technique in patients with prostate cancer. Int J Radiat Oncol Biol Phys 48:649–656
90. Chao KS, Lin M (2002) Lymphangiogram-assisted lymph node target delineation for patients with gynecologic malignancies. Int J Radiat Oncol Biol Phys 54:1147–1152
91. Portaluri M, Bambace S, Perez C et al (2004) Clinical and anatomical guidelines in pelvic cancer contouring for radiotherapy treatment planning. Cancer Radiother 8:222–229
92. Portaluri M, Bambace S, Perez C, Angone G (2005) A three-dimensional definition of nodal spaces on the basis of CT images showing enlarged nodes for pelvic radiotherapy. Int J Radiat Oncol Biol Phys 63:1101–1107
93. Workmanns D, Diederich S, Lentschig MG, Winter F, Heindel W (2000) Spiral CT of pulmonary nodules: interobserver variation in assessment of lesion size. Eur Radiol 10:710–713
94. Armstrong J, McGibney C (2000) The impact of three-dimensional radiation on the treatment of non-small cell lung cancer. Radiother Oncol 56:157–167

95. Lagerwaard FJ, Van Sornsen de Koste JR, Nijssen-Visser MR et al (2001) Multiple "slow" CT scans for in corporating lung tumor mobility in radiotherapy planning. Int J Radiat Oncol Biol Phys 51:932–937
96. Harris KM, Adams H, Lloyd DC, Harvey DJ (1993) The effect on apparent size of simulated pulmonary nodules of using three standard CT window settings. Clin Radiol 47:241–244
97. Giraud P (2000) Influence of CT images visualization parameters for target volume delineation in lung cancer. Proceedings of 19th ESTRO Istanbul, 2000. Radiother Oncol S39
98. Halperin EC, Schmidt-Ullrich RK, Perez CA, Brady LW (2004) Overview and basic science of radiation oncology. In: Perez CA, Brady LW, Halperin EC, Schmidt-Ullrich RK (eds) Principles and practice of radiation oncology. Lippincott Williams and Wilkins, Baltimore, pp 1–95
99. Levitt SH, Perez CA, Hui S, Purdy JA (2008) Evolution of computerized radiation therapy in radiation oncology: potential problems and solutions. Int J Radiat Oncol Bio Phys 70:978–986
100. Ling CC, Humm J, Larson S et al (2000) Towards multidimensional radiotherapy (MD-3D CRT): biological imaging and biological conformality. Int J Radiat Oncol Biol Phys 47:551–560
101. Roach M, Faillace-Akazawa P, Malfatti C, Holland J, Hricak H (1996) Prostate volumes defined by magnetic resonance imaging and computerized tomographic scans for three-dimensional conformal radiotherapy. Int J Radiat Oncol Biol Phys 35:1011–1018
102. Mullerad M, Hricak H, Wang L et al (2004) Prostate cancer: detection of extracapsular extension by genitourinary and general radiologists at MR imaging. Radiology 232:140–146
103. Keall P (2004) 4-dimensional computed tomography imaging and treatment planning. Semin Radiat Oncol 14:81–90
104. Gierga DP, Chen GT, Kung JH et al (2004) Quantification of respiration-induced abdominal tumor motion and its impact on IMRT dose distributions. Int J Radiat Oncol Biol Phys 58:1584–1595
105. Langen KM, Jones DTL (2001) Organ motion and its management. Int J Radiat Oncol Biol Phys 50:265–278
106. Rosenzweig KE, Yorke E, Amols H et al (2005) Tumor motion control in the treatment of non-small cell lung cancer. Cancer Invest 23:129–133
107. Sheng K, Molloy JA, Read PW (2006) Intensity-modulated radiation therapy (IMRT) dosimetry of the head and neck: a comparison of treatment plans using linear accelerator-based IMRT and helical tomotherapy. Int J Radiat Oncol Biol Phys 65:917–923
108. Shih HA, Harisinghani M, Zietman AL et al (2005) Mapping of nodal disease in locally advanced prostate cancer: rethinking the clinical target volume for pelvic nodal irradiation based on vascular rather than bony anatomy. Int J Radiat Oncol Biol Phys 63:1262–1269
109. Allen AM, Siracuse KM, Hayman JA et al (2004) Evaluation of the influence of breathing on the movement and modeling of lung tumors. Int J Radiat Oncol Biol Phys 58:1251–1257
110. Herman MG (2005) Clinical use of electronic portal imaging. Semin Radiat Oncol 15:157–167
111. Weltens C, Menten J, Feron M et al (2001) Interobserver variations in gross tumor volume delineation of brain tumors on computed tomography and impact of magnetic resonance imaging. Radiother Oncol 60:49–59
112. Leunens G, Menten J, Weltens C, Verstraete J, van der Schueren E (1993) Quality assessment of medical decision making in radiation oncology: variability in target volume delineation for brain tumors. Radiother Oncol 29:169–175

References

113. Ten Haken RK, Thornton AF, Sandler HM et al (1992) A quantitative assessment of the addition of MRI to CT-based, 3-D treatment planning of brain tumors. Radiother Oncol 25:121–133
114. Rasch C, Barillot I, Remeijer P, Touw A, van Herk M, Lebesque JV (1999) Definition of the prostate in CT and MRI: A multi-observer study. Int J Radiat Oncol Biol Phys 43:57–66
115. Rasch C, Keus R, Pameijer FA et al (1997) The potential impact of CT-MRI matching on tumor volume delineation in advanced head and neck cancer. Int J Radiat Oncol Biol Phys 39:841–848
116. Caldwell CB, Mah K, Skinner M, Danjoux CE (2003) Can PET provide the 3D extent of tumor motion for individualized internal target volumes? A phantom study of the limitations of CT and the promise of PET. Int J Radiat Oncol Biol Phys 55:1381–1393
117. Chapman JD, Bradley JD, Eary JF et al (2003) Molecular (functional) imaging for radiotherapy applications: an RTOG symposium. Int J Radiat Oncol Biol Phys 55:294–301
118. Munley MT, Marks LB, Hardenbergh PH, Bentel GC (2001) Functional imaging of normal tissues with nuclear medicine: applications in radiotherapy. Semin Radiat Oncol 11:28–36
119. Grosu AL, Piert M, Weber WA et al (2005) Positron emission tomography for radiation treatment planning. Strahlenther Onkol 181:483–499
120. Paulino AC, Koshy M, Howell R et al (2005) Comparison of CT- and FDG-PET-defined gross tumor volume in intensity-modulated radiotherapy for head-and-neck cancer. Int J Radiat Oncol Biol Phys 61:1385–1392
121. Gregoire V (2004) Is there any future in radiotherapy planning without the use of PET: unraveling the myth. Radiother Oncol 73:261–263
122. Bourguet P, Groupe de Travail SOR (2003) Standards, options and recommendations 2002 for the use of positron emission tomography with [18F] FDG (PET FDG) in cancerology (integral connection). Bull Cancer S5–S17
123. Caldwell CB, Mah K, Ung YC et al (2001) Observer variation in contouring gross tumor volume in patients with poorly defined non-small cell lung tumors on CT: the impact of 18FDG-Hybrid PET fusion. Int J Radiat Oncol Biol Phys 51:923–931
124. Chao KSC, Bosch WR, Mutic S et al (2001) A novel approach to overcome hypoxic tumor resistance: Cu-ATSM-guided intensity-modulated radiation therapy. Int J Radiat Oncol Biol Phys 49:1171–1182
125. Hill DLG, Batchelor PG, Holden M, Hawkes DJ (2001) Medical image registration. Phys Med Biol 46:R1–R45
126. Mutic S, Dempsey JF, Bosch WR et al (2001) Multimodality image registration quality assurance for conformal three-dimensional treatment planning. Int J Radiat Oncol Biol Phys 51:244–260
127. Rosenman J (2001) Incorporating functional imaging information into radiation treatment. Semin Radiat Oncol 11:83–92
128. Pelizzari CA, Lujan AE (2005) Imaging and fusion technologies. In: Mundt AJ, Roeske JC (eds) Intensity modulated radiation therapy: a clinical perspective. Decker, Toronto
129. Rosenman JG, Miller EP, Tracton G, Cullip TJ (1998) Image registration: an essential part of radiation therapy treatment planning. Int J Radiat Oncol Biol Phys 40:197–205
130. Balter JM, Lam K, Sandler HM, Littles JF, Bree RL, Ten Haken RK (1995) Measurement of prostate movement over the course of routine radiotherapy using implanted markers. Int J Radiat Oncol Biol Phys 31:113–118

131. Roach M, Faillace-Akazawa P, Malfatti C (1997) Prostate volumes and organ movements defined by serial computerized tomographic scans during three-dimensional conformal radiotherapy. Radiat Oncol Invest 5:187–194
132. Tinger A, Michalski JM, Cheng A et al (1998) A critical evaluation of the planning target volume for 3-D conformal radiotherapy of prostate cancer. Int J Radiat Oncol Biol Phys 42:213–221
133. van Herk M, Bruce A, Kroes APG, Shouman T, Touw A, Lebesque JV (1995) Quantification of organ motion during conformal radiotherapy of the prostate by three dimensional image registration. Int J Radiat Oncol Biol Phys 33:1311–1320
134. Balter JM, Lam KL, McGinn CJ et al (1998) Improvement of CT-based treatment-planning models of abdominal targets using static exhale imaging. Int J Radiat Oncol Biol Phys 41:939–943
135. Hanley J, Debois MM, Mah D et al (1999) Deep inspiration breath-hold technique for lung tumors: the potential value of target immobilization and reduced lung density in dose escalation. Int J Radiat Oncol Biol Phys 45:603–611
136. Bedford JL, Shentall GS (1998) A digital method for computing target margins in radiotherapy. Med Phys 25:224–231
137. Antolak JA, Rosen IL (1999) Planning target volumes for radiotherapy: how much margin is needed. Int J Radiat Oncol Biol Phys 44:1165–1170
138. van Herk M, Remeijer P, Rasch C, Lebesque JV (2000) The probability of correct target dosage: dose-population histograms for deriving treatment margins in radiotherapy. Int J Radiat Oncol Biol Phys 47:1121–1135
139. Craig T, Battista J, Moisennko V, Van Dyk J (2001) Considerations for the implementation of target volume protocols in radiation therapy. Int J Radiat Oncol Biol Phys 49:241–250
140. van Herk M, Remeijer P, Lebesque JV (2002) Inclusion of geometric uncertainties in treatment plan evaluations. Int J Radiat Oncol Biol Phys 52:1407–1422
141. Yu CX, Jaffray DA, Wong JW (1998) The effects of intra-fraction organ motion on the delivery of dynamic intensity modulation. Phys Med Biol 43:91–104
142. Kubo HD, Wang L (2000) Compatibility of Varian 2100C gated operations with enhanced dynamic wedge and IMRT dose delivery. Med Phys 27:1732–1737
143. Shimizu S, Shirato H, Ogura S et al (2001) Detection of lung tumor movement in real-time tumor-tracking radiotherapy. Int J Radiat Oncol Biol Phys 51:304–310
144. Bortfeld T, Jokivarsi K, Goitein M, Kung J, Jiang SB (2002) Effects of intra-fraction motion on IMRT dose delivery: statistical analysis and simulation. Phys Med Biol 47:2203–2220
145. Lattanzi J, McNeeley S, Pinover W et al (1999) A comparison of daily CT localization to a daily ultrasound-based system in prostate cancer. Int J Radiat Oncol Biol Phys 43:719–725
146. Onishi H, Kuriyama K, Komiyama T et al (2004) Clinical outcomes of stereotactic radiotherapy for stage I non-small cell lung cancer using a novel irradiation technique: patient self-controlled breath-hold and beam switching using a combination linear accelerator and CT scanner. Lung Cancer 45:45–55
147. Rosenzweig KE, Hanley J, Mah D et al (2000) The deep inspiration breath-hold technique in the treatment of inoperable non-small-cell lung cancer. Int J Radiat Oncol Biol Phys 48:81–87
148. Wong J, Sharpe M, Jaffray D et al (1999) The use of active breathing control (ABC) to reduce margin for breathing control. Int J Radiat Oncol Biol Phys 44:911–919

149. Yan D, Ziaga E, Jaffray D (1998) The use of adaptive radiation therapy to reduce setup error: a prospective clinical study. Int J Radiat Oncol Biol Phys 41:715–720
150. Yan D, Lockman D, Brabbins D, Tyburski L, Martinez A (2000) An off-line strategy for constructing a patient-specific planning target volume in adaptive treatment process for prostate cancer. Int J Radiat Oncol Biol Phys 48:289–302
151. Yan D, Lockman D (2001) Organ/patient geometric variation in external beam radiotherapy and its effects. Med Phys 28:593–602
152. Purdy JA, Vijayakumar S, Perez CA, Levitt SH (2006) Physics of treatment planning in radiation oncology. In: Levitt SH, Purdy JA, Perez CA, Vijayakumar S (eds) Technical basis of radiation therapy: practical clinical applications, 4th revised edn. Springer, Berlin, pp 69–106
153. Bussels B, Hermans R, Reijnders A et al (2006) Retropharyngeal lymph nodes in squamous cell carcinoma of oropharynx: incidence, localization, and implications for target volume. Int J Radiat Oncol Biol Phys 65:733–738
154. Braam PM, Raaijmakers CPJ, Terhaard CHJ (2007) Cranial location of level II lymph nodes in laryngeal cancer: implications for elective nodal target volume delineation. Int J Radiat Oncol Biol Phys 67:462–468
155. Prins-Braam P, Raaijmakers CPJ, Terhaard CHJ (2004) Location of cervical lymph node metastases in oropharyngeal and hypopharyngeal carcinoma: implications for cranial border of elective nodal target volumes. Int J Radiat Oncol Biol Phys 58:132–138
156. Yuan S, Meng X, Yu J et al (2007) Determining optimal clinical target volume margins on the basis of microscopic extracapsular extension of metastatic nodes in patients with non-small cell lung cancer. Int J Radiat Oncol Biol Phys 67:727–734
157. Steenbakkers RJHM, Fitton JCDI, Deurloo KEI et al (2006) Reduction of observer variation using matched CT-PET for lung cancer delineation: a three-dimensional analysis. Int J Radiat Oncol Biol Phys 64:435–448
158. Ashamalla H, Rafla S, Parikh K et al (2005) The contribution of integrated PET/CT to the evolving definition of treatment volumes in radiation treatment planning in lung cancer. Int J Radiat Oncol Biol Phys 63:1016–1023
159. Bradley J, Thorstad WL, Mutic S et al (2004) Impact of FDG-PET on radiation therapy volume delineation in non-small-cell lung cancer. Int J Radiat Oncol Biol Phys 59:78–86
160. Brunner TB, Merkel S, Grabenbauer GG et al (2005) Definition of elective lymphatic target volume in ductal carcinoma of the pancreatic head based on histopathological analysis. Int J Radiat Oncol Biol Phys 62:1021–1029
161. Campostrini F, Gragianin M, Rampin L et al (2002) How iliopelvic lymphoscintigraphy can affect the definition of planning target volume in radiation therapy of pelvic and testicular tumors. Int J Radiat Oncol Biol Phys 53:1303–1313
162. Finlay MH, Ackerman I, Tirona RG et al (2006) Use of CT simulation for treatment of cervical cancer to assess the adequacy of lymph node coverage of conventional pelvic fields based on bony landmarks. Int J Radiat Oncol Biol Phys 64:205–209
163. Guckenberg M, Meyer J, Vordermark D et al (2006) Magnitude and clinical relevance of translational and rotational patient setup errors: a cone-beam CT study. Int J Radiat Oncol Biol Phys 65:934–942
164. Oelfke U, Tucking T, Nill S et al (2006) Linac-integrated kV-cone beam CT: technical features and first applications. Med Dosim 31:62–70

165. Pouliot J, Bani-Hashemi A, Chen J et al (2005) Low-dose megavoltage cone-beam CT for radiation therapy. Int J Radiat Oncol Biol Phys 62:552–650
166. Jeraj R, Mackie TR, Balog J et al (2004) Radiation characteristics of helical tomotherapy. Med Phys 31:396–404
167. Mackie TR, Holmes TW, Swerdloff S et al (1993) Tomotherapy: a new concept for the delivery of conformal radiotherapy. Med Phys 20:1709–1719
168. Shirato H, Shimizu S, Kunieda T, et al (2000) Physical aspects of a real-time tumor-tracking system for gated radiotherapy. Int J Radiat Oncol Biol Phys 48:1187–1195
169. Mell LK, Mehrotra AK, Mundt AJ (2005) Intensity-modulated radiation therapy use in United States, 2004. Cancer 104:1296–1303
170. Simpson JR, Dryzmala RE, Rich KM (2006) Stereotactic radiosurgery and radiotherapy. In: Levitt SH, Purdy JA, Perez CA, Vijayakumar S (eds) Technical basis of radiation therapy: practical clinical applications, 4th revised edn. Springer, Berlin, pp 203–253
171. Ramsey CR, Langen KM, Kupelian PA et al (2006) A technique for adaptive image-guided helical tomotherapy for lung cancer. Int J Radiat Oncol Biol Phys 64:1237–1244
172. Hodge W, Tome WA, Jaradat HA et al (2006) Feasibility report of image guided stereotactic body radiotherapy (IG-SBRT) with tomotherapy for early stage medically inoperable lung cancer using extreme hypofractionation. Acta Oncol 45:890–896
173. Antonuk L (2002) Electronic portal imaging devices: a review and historical perspective of contemporary technologies and research. Phys Med Biol 47:R31–R65
174. Erridge SC, Seppenwoolde Y, Muller SH et al (2003) Portal imaging to assess setup-errors, tumor motion and tumor shrinkage during conformal radiotherapy of non-small cell lung cancer. Radiother Oncol 66:75–85
175. Scarbrough TJ, Golden NM, Ting JY et al (2006) Comparison of ultrasound and implanted seed marker prostate localization methods: implications for image-guided radiotherapy. Int J Radiat Oncol Biol Phys 65:378–387
176. Hall E (2006) Intensity modulated radiation therapy, protons and risk of second cancers. Int J Radiat Oncol Biol Phys 65:1–7
177. Aoyama H, Wisterly BS, Mackie TR et al (2006) Integral radiation dose to normal structures with conformal external beam radiation. Int J Radiat Oncol Biol Phys 64:962–967
178. BIPM: Bureau International des Poids et Mesures. Recommendation R(I)-1 in BIPM Com. Cons. Etalons Mes. Ray. Ionisants (Section I). (Offilib, F-75240 Paris Cedex 05): R(I)15
179. Court L, Rosen I, Mohan R et al (2003) Evaluation of mechanical precision and alignment uncertainties for an integrated CT/linac system. Med Phys 30:1–13
180. IMRT CWG, NCI IMRT Collaborative Working Group (2001) Intensity modulated radiation therapy: current status and issues of interest. Int J Radiat Oncol Biol Phys 51:880–914
181. Kutcher GJ, Coia L, Gillin M et al (1994) Comprehensive QA for radiation oncology report of AAPM Radiation Therapy Committee Task Group 40. Med Phys 21:581–618
182. Low DA, Lu W, Purdy JA, Perez CA, Levitt SH (2006) Intensity-modulated radiation therapy. In: Levitt SH, Purdy JA, Perez CA, Vijayakumar S (eds) Technical basis of radiation therapy: practical clinical applications, 4th revised edn. Springer, Berlin, pp 203–231
183. Mohan R, Low D, Chao KSC et al (2004) Intensity modulated radiation treatment planning quality assurance, delivery and clinical application. In: Perez CA, Brady LW, Halperin

EC, Schmidt-Ulrich RK (eds) Principles and practice of radiation oncology, 4th edn. Lippincott, Williams and Wilkins, Baltimore, pp 314–336
184. Poortmans PM et al (2005) The quality assurance program of the Radiotherapy Group of the European Organization for Research and Treatment of Cancer: past, present and future. Eur J Surg Oncol 31:667–674
185. Purdy JA (2004) Three-dimensional conformal radiation therapy: physics, treatment planning and clinical aspects. In: Perez CA, Brady LW, Halperin EC, Schmidt-Ulrich RK (eds) Principles and practice of radiation oncology, 4th edn. Lippincott, Williams and Wilkins, Baltimore, pp 283–313
186. Purdy JA, Harms WB, Matthews JW et al (1993) Advances in 3-dimensional radiation treatment planning systems: room-view display with real time interactivity. Int J Radiat Oncol Biol Phys 27:933–944
187. Perez CA et al (1997) Cost benefit of emerging technology in localized carcinoma of the prostate. Int J Radiat Oncol Biol Phys 39:875–883
188. Pollack A, Zagars GK, Starkschall G et al (2002) Prostate cancer radiation dose response: results of the M D Anderson phase III randomized trial. Int J Radiat Oncol Biol Phys 53:1097–1105
189. Suit H (2002) The Gray lecture 2001: coming technical advances in radiation oncology. Int J Radiat Oncol Biol Phys 53:798–809

Printing and Binding: Stürtz GmbH, Würzburg